Comparative Public Policy and Citizen Participation

Pergamon Policy Studies on Politics and Administration

Hadley   *Split Ticket Voting in America*
Miller, Suchner & Voelker   *Citizenship in an Age of Science*
Perry & Angle   *Labor Relations and Public Agency Effectiveness*

Related Titles

Coppock & Sewell   *The Spatial Dimensions of Public Policy*
Foxley, Aninat & Arellano   *Redistributive Effects on Government
   Programmes: The Chilean Case*
Segall   *Human Behavior and Public Policy*

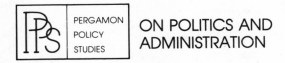

PERGAMON POLICY STUDIES

ON POLITICS AND ADMINISTRATION

Comparative Public Policy and Citizen Participation

Energy, Education,
Health and Urban Issues in
the U.S. and Germany

Edited by
Charles R. Foster

Pergamon Press
NEW YORK • OXFORD • TORONTO • SYDNEY • FRANKFURT • PARIS

Pergamon Press Offices:

U.S.A. Pergamon Press Inc., Maxwell House, Fairview Park, Elmsford, New York 10523, U.S.A.

U.K. Pergamon Press Ltd., Headington Hill Hall, Oxford OX3 0BW, England

CANADA Pergamon of Canada, Ltd., 150 Consumers Road, Willowdale, Ontario M2J, 1P9, Canada

AUSTRALIA Pergamon Press (Aust) Pty. Ltd., P O Box 544, Potts Point, NSW 2011, Australia

FRANCE Pergamon Press SARL, 24 rue des Ecoles, 75240 Paris, Cedex 05, France

FEDERAL REPUBLIC OF GERMANY Pergamon Press GmbH, 6242 Kronberg/Taunus, Pferdstrasse 1, Federal Republic of Germany

Library of Congress Cataloging in Publication Data

International Conference on Participation and Policy-
  Making, Politische Akademie Tutzing, 1978.
  Comparative public policy and citizen participation.

  (Pergamon policy studies)
  "Jointly sponsored by the Bonn University Center
for Political Participation and the Conference Group
on German Politics."
  Bibliography: p.
  Includes index.
  1. Political participation—United States—Con-
gresses. 2. Political participation—Germany, West—
Congresses. I. Foster, Charles R., 1927-
II. Bonn. Universitat. Studiengruppe Partizi-
pationsforschung. III. Conference Group on German
Politics. IV. Title.
JK1764.I57 1978   351'.8   79-20377
ISBN 0-08-024624-9

Printed in the United States of America

Contents

Acknowledgments

The papers in this volume are based on a German-American conference on participation and politics held at Tutzing, Bavaria, June 5-9, 1978. The conference was jointly sponsored by the Bonn University Center for Political Participation and the Conference Group on German Politics, (CGGP) an independent organization of scholars devoted to the study of German affairs. It was hosted by the Akademie fur Politische Bildung, Tutzing, Bavaria.

The intent of this book is to present views of German and American scholars on relationships between participation and policy making. It is difficult to take a number of papers, no matter how excellent, that were given at an international conference and to make a book out of them. Fortunately, my task has been eased by the willingness of the authors to make extensive revisions of the articles. I have thus been able to provide a design that divides up the book into separate sections.

I am grateful for the hospitality and support of Professor Manfred Hattich, Director of the Political Academy in Tutzing, which is on the shore of beautiful Lake Starnberg in Bavaria. The Chairman of the Conference, Professor Alfred Diamant, of Indiana University steadfastly encouraged my work on this book. I want to thank also William Glaser, Arnold Heidenheimer, Bruce Smith, and Horst Zillessen for their continued active interest. CGGP Chairman George Romoser, Professor of Political Science at the University of New Hampshire, and Dr. D. Brent Smith of Washington, D.C. were instrumental in organizing the Tuzting Conference from the American side and securing travel and conference funding. I also wish to thank Richard Rowson, Gwen Bell, and Angela Clark of Pergamon Press for their ready counsel. My wife, whose support and forbearance were steadfast, helped with the

editing.   John   Packman   of   Princeton   University   provided
additional   editorial   assistance,   as   did   Stephen   Artner,
Daniel Hamilton, David Long, and Anne Vorce.

Introduction

Demand has been rising in all quarters for more popular involvement in policy formulation. Participation is often seen as a cure for the alienation and sense of individual impotence widely experienced in postindustrial societies. At the same time, new styles and modalities of participation are required if the implementation of desired policies is to be more effective.

While participation has been a central issue in political science since Plato and Aristotle, public policy is a rather more recent concern. Inquiry into the processes of policy production and the contents of government policies is largely a recent phenomenon. In this volume, both participation and policy outputs are treated in a comparative fashion through both normative and empirical lines of inquiry. After attempting to determine which groups and individuals participate in the various aspects of the policy process, the authors of these articles inquire whether the existing participatory patterns should be preserved or whether they should examine alternative models.

The discussion centers around four basic issues crucial to the future of Western societies. Energy, an increasingly scarce and expensive commodity, is essential for economic growth and stability, yet concern for the environment and fear of nuclear power breed conflict at both the elite and popular levels. In the field of education - in an age of almost universal literacy, instant communication, and widespread technical specialization - there is growing pressure from teachers, students, and parents regarding the style and content of instruction. Municipal policy, traditionally the locus of direct citizen involvement, is being revitalized in many areas by increasing popular awareness, but participation in the making of such policy is constrained by expanding and often ill-defined national and provincial jurisdictions. Health care, of vital concern to every individual, is directly affected by governmental action but is still largely immune to direct popular pressures and initiatives. In each of these four areas, established political processes have only begun to respond to demands for greater participation in policy formulation and execution.

Before the articles that discuss these four issues there are two contributions that examine a phenomenon symptomatic of the demand for wider participation in numerous areas: the citizens' action movement that has emerged in West Germany since the late 1960s. After outlining the development, scope, and principal causes of this movement, Uwe Thaysen and Stephen Artner explain the salient characteristics of the German citizens' action groups. In particular, the authors examine the groups' attitudes, objectives, and contributions to the German constitutional and political system. Finally, they focus on the probable future development of this mode of popular participation in light of the increasingly tangled jurisdictions of federal, local, and provincial authorities. Horst Zillessen argues that the German citizens' action movement reveals structural flaws of current representative democracy, in which bureaucratic executive authority expands into private and social areas at the expense of the authority of elected legislative bodies. Suggesting that a widely felt dissatisfaction with the state is in reality discontent with the existing parties, Zillessen considers the new opportunities for participation in energy and environmental policy provided by federal law and "planning cells" and then presents a new organizational model for participation of local citizens.

Three contributions deal with participation in the energy policy area. Heino Galland begins by contrasting numerous demands for participation with the inadequate participatory opportunities in this field. He pays particular attention to the structure of the energy-policy field as compared with that of traditional participatory domains and checks existing models of participation against practical experience. Galland predicts that challenging entrenched technocratic influences by verifiable but noninstitutionalized forms of participation can only result in continued conflict over participation and public policy. Joan Aron examines the financial costs citizens' groups incur in hiring specialists to take part in highly technical debates over energy policy. She explores the legal and administrative implications of government funding of responsible citizens' groups. Intervenor funding, which is gaining acceptance in the American executive branch and Congress, has become increasingly feasible as agencies involved with energy issues come to recognize the valuable contributions provided by greater citizen participation. Michael Pollak then focuses on the style and content of the German antinuclear movement, revealing the ambiguous response to the new citizen activism by liberals, conservatives, and the radical left. After tracing the movement's origins to the rapid social and economic change of the postwar era, Pollak considers the value of this ambiguity in maintaining the unity and tactical flexibility of the ideologically diverse members of the antinuclear movement. He says that the avoidance of full integration in German institutions may be a strength rather than a weakness of the antinuclear groups.

Following this discussion of energy issues, four papers deal with participation in the field of education, where the debate takes a quite different form. Here, suggests Maurice Garnier, one must first reexamine the decisive role of the educational bureaucracy, for a number of societal characteristics require that education be bureaucratically managed. Garnier then raises the question of coordination between organizations, introducing the notion of "loosely coupled" structures and inquiring whether German organizational forms might not be applicable to other countries. Robert Salisbury considers the special place participation occupies in American education, where the issue of its role mirrors the larger question of whether the state arises from popular participation, as the Lockean tradition assumes. Salisbury examines the forms, purposes, and degree of participation in actual educational policy making in a study of six St. Louis school districts. He then relates individual motivation to institutional context in a theoretical discussion of the differing objectives pursued in varying institutional arenas.

In contrast to the American participation in educational policy making, participation in the West German educational system has no definite place, as is demonstrated in Raimund Klauser's discussion of participatory demands in continuing-education programs for German teachers. Participation is shown to be an innovation in the highly centralized German educational system, but its development must be a learning process if present institutional structures are to be preserved. Treating another aspect of German education, Wulf Drexler describes the history and organization of a recent educational experiment, the Oberstufen-Kolleg attached to the new "reform university" of Bielefeld. The experiment has revealed something of the complexity of participatory innovation in an educational bureaucracy that includes teachers themselves as state officials.

Local politics provides a locus of direct participation in the form of voting, campaigning, testifying, lobbying, demonstrating, and petitioning municipal officials. Gordon P. Whitaker discusses such efforts as they are directed at the delivery of "human services" - activities such as education, health care, and crisis intervention, which are designed to affect individuals directly, rather then their physical or socioeconomic environments. In areas where "raw material,"

"consumer," and "finished product" all refer to the same
party, the citizen must assume a direct responsibility for
public policy, and the sometimes hazy distinction between
cooperation and coercion takes on added importance. Prodosh
Aich addresses the problems of participation in local government in general; he says that there is a crisis in democracy
as parliamentary systems become increasingly aware of citizens
at the local level. Departing from traditional analysis, Aich
seeks to develop an approach to participation research that
draws its general principles from concrete descriptions of the
interests at work in local politics. The author pays particular
attention to the conflicts between local and national interests
and those between elected officials and administrative
specialists. Finally, in a Marxist interpretation of the participation debate, Adalbert Evers and Juan Rodriguez-Lores
discuss established state institutions and processes in relation
to opposing economic classes which seek to establish their own
social and cultural hegemony. Drawing on Gramsci's analysis
as well as on German socialist tradition, the authors suggest
that the rise of urban protest movements in Italy and France
could have serious implications for participation in the Federal
Republic.

A final group of contributions discuss participation in the
vital field of health care. Christa Altenstetter provides a
context for this discussion by comparing health-policy processes in West Germany and the United States. She demonstrates that modes of participation must vary according to
the specific policy-making structures involved. Lawrence
Brown goes on to furnish an overview of federal health policy
formulation in the United States. He argues that the federal
government has intervened in the medical field with a series of
strategies each of which emerges in response to the flaws of
its predecessors. Each policy departure effort is based upon
a distinct rationale and a particular political coalition, and a
knowledge of both is essential to an understanding of federal
behavior in the health-care field. In a case study of American
medical policy, Virginia Cohn Parkum examines the participatory opportunities established by the comprehensive health
planning legislation of 1966. An important feature of this
legislation was the establishment of area councils to provide
comprehensive planning for their respective regions. Parkum
discusses the composition of these councils, the motivations of
their members, the regulations under which they operate, and
the amount of participation that has actually taken place.

The authors of this book exhibit widely varying concerns,
approaches, and points of view. They raise myriad questions
about popular participation and public policy, only a few of
which can receive detailed attention. Yet despite their differing outlooks and conclusions, the contributors to this
volume agree on the growing significance of participatory

demands in the United States and the Federal Republic of Germany. Participation can take many forms and pursue many goals, but it cannot be long impeded or suppressed in democratic states. Rather, in the decade ahead it can and must contribute to the political, social, and economic well-being of the industrialized West.

I

Policy Making in the United States and Germany

1 Analyzing United States Policy Making
Robert A. Levine

Modern policy analysis, with roots in economics and systems analysis, has been in conscious use within the United States government for almost twenty years - since Secretary of Defense Robert McNamara and his "whiz kids" came to the Pentagon. Its intellectual roots go back to the operations analysis of the Second World War.

However, only in the last decade has the recognition grown that policy analysis must depend strongly on the policy-making structure itself as well as on the structure to which the analysis is applied. McNamara and his minions, for example, were far less effective than they might have been because they never came to grips with the role of the United States Congress in making defense policy. On the other hand, they were far more effective in making fundamental change than has sometimes been realized because they altered the institutional structure of defense policy making by forcing the military services to promote in their own self-interest the kind of officers and civilians who could cope with the whiz kids.

During the 1970s, the American style of policy analysis has been spreading through the Western world, less because of American evangelism than because of the needs of other nations. The coincidence, however, of these two movements - the recognition of the dependence of policy analysis upon policy-making structure and the international spread of analysis - has not led to much adaptation of United States analysis to foreign forms. This has caused some misunderstanding. The U.S. Congressional Budget Office (CBO), for example, has achieved in three years a reputation for effective analytical assistance to the Congress, and, as a result, delegations of parliamentarians from other Western democracies occasionally visit CBO to ask how they might benefit from the advantages the Congress gets from its new policy-analysis installation. The answer, unfortunately, is that they probably cannot. The Congress is a major maker of American policy, sometimes substantially outweighing the President himself, and policy analysis that assists Congressional policy making can therefore be effective policy analysis. However, all other Western parliaments are, to a greater or lesser degree, instruments whose primary function is to choose a government and, except in the most exceptional circumstances, to ratify the government's decisions. Devices such as the "question period" in the House of Commons do help keep the government accountable to parliament and the electorate, but they give parliament little power over policy direction, not to mention detail. Policy analysis for such bodies under such circumstances runs the risk of being rather sterile.

Democratic governments are enough alike, however, that policy analysis for such governments deals with broad areas of shared characteristics. One category that includes many of the common attributes of democracies is pluralism, that is, the working of multiple influences in the making of policy. The existence of pluralism means that no government will arrive at a set of policies purely or even primarily through analysis. Good analysis, though, may have an effect on policies through one or more channels. If policy analysis is to be effective, it must take account of this pluralism, include it in its analysis, and understand how best to express the analysis under a pluralistic regime.

This stress on pluralism is important for democratic countries in general because many interests and views exert influence on policy through many channels. Beyond that, the similarity of democracies begins to break down. The United States is more complex than most. Some of the reasons for this are well understood: the United States is the Western world's largest democracy; it also has a federal system which, although it is not unique, differs somewhat from most other Western democracies.

The crucial difference between the United States and all other Western democracies, however, is the constitutional structure that magnifies and institutionalizes pluralism: policy-making power is divided between the executive and legislative branches of government, with the legislative branch being divided into two equally powerful independent houses. (The third branch, the independent judiciary, is less relevant here because in principle it reviews policy rather than makes it.)

The complexity of the United States policy-making system exacerbates the difficulties in understanding how policy is made and how policy analysis can be used. The four examples discussed in this paper are peculiar to the United States. These political events examined here could not have occurred the same way in other nations, and thus policy analysis could

not have played the same role. Policy analysis of the events
must therefore demonstrate an understanding of this role.
     The basic model for analysis is based on the pluralism
that characterizes all democracies, and, even more fundamentally, on a feature common to all governments, whether democratic or not. This universal feature is the tension in the
making of policy between the interpretation of public or
common interest and efforts of various special or partial
interests to improve their positions and to bargain over the
distribution of outcomes.
     The definitions of the common interest or the public
interest (used interchangeably here) and of partial interests or
special interests are of key importance, particularly because
they are easily misunderstood. (What is not meant is a
Manichaean attribution of "common interest" or "partial
interests" to different people or groups with emphasis on good
versus evil.) Indeed, this is one of the points: groups come
to policy decisions in varying ways in varying situations, and
individuals mix the two kinds of interest in their own thinking
about policy. The distinction is in between the different ways
of influencing policy events. The common interest influences
events through arguments, contending that the position taken
is preferable for a majority or an organic entity greater than
any individual or specific group. As Richard Flathman says,

> The logic of the concept will always allow us to ask
> "Why is that policy in the public interest?" The
> answer, "Because individual or group X regards it
> as in his or its interest," will never be responsive
> to that question.(1)

     Partial or special interests, as the terms are used here,
deal explicitly with what is good for them. By the use of
political power, collective bargaining, or whatever power is
available to them, they attempt to increase their ration of
power or resources. Events are influenced and policy is
made in both these ways, and it is a matter of concern to
policy analysis how the two modes mix and how they may be
affected by analysis.
     Private analysis itself deals with the first part of this
model. In order to influence public policy (policy analysis can
also influence private policy, in which case the good of,
e.g., the firm or the party may be substituted for the common
good) analysts attempt to determine the common interest, to
find a rational solution that maximizes the common interest as
it is viewed by those making policy decisions, and to convince
the decision makers by using analytical common-interest
arguments rather than their own bargaining power.
     One standard explanation of policy making in the United
States, however, denies that policy analysts' rational solutions

are likely to influence policy. The contentions are that the distribution of power and resources is the key question in policy making, that such distribution is ordinarily affected by bargaining, and that bargaining leads to outcomes preferable to those imposed in the name of the common interest or a rational solution designed by policy analysts.

The construct used to describe national policy making in this line of argument is the key triangle that exists in any policy area (e.g., defense, health, education) and that consists of an inside bureaucracy, an outside interest group, and interested Congressional committees. Emphasizing mutual interests and eliminating competing ones, these components combine to push legislation. This construct helps describe many situations, but it has two major shortcomings. First, it gives almost no weight to the relevance of common-interest arguments, manifesting an extreme degree of skepticism about rationality and public interest in the policy-making process which is not justified. As is suggested above and illustrated by the examples discussed below, common-interest rationality is a strand in public decision making, and well-conceived policy analysis can increase its role. Second, the triangle model fails to explain that even inside the decision-making process of individuals - Presidents, bureaucrats, and Congressmen, for example - views of the public interest and narrower interests play roles that vary according to circumstances.

Some of this abstract discussion may be clarified by the following examples of policy making in four United States cases: "maximum feasible participation" of the poor in the poverty programs, federal aid to education, welfare reform, and energy conservation. The first two of these policies have been enacted; as yet, the last two have not.

"MAXIMUM FEASIBLE PARTICIPATION"
OF THE POOR IN POVERTY PROGRAMS

"Maximum feasible participation" is the phrase under which management of many poverty programs, particularly the local ones, of President Lyndon Johnson's "War on Poverty" during the late 1960s were turned over in part or entirely to the intended beneficiaries.

The contention that effects of this form of participation were favorable is controversial, but it may be less controversial than whether the authors of the "maximum feasible participation" concept even intended for it to produce favorable results. Daniel Moynihan, one of the authors of the legislation, claims that no more was intended than a gesture toward listening to those who would be affected by the programs.(2) Others, though, intended it to imply that the major degree of control was to be transferred to program beneficiaries, as frequently happened.

What apparently happened was that various social theorists of the early 1960s, particularly those associated with the Juvenile Delinquency program of the Kennedy Department of Justice and the Ford Foundation's "Grey Areas" program, promoted the idea of the necessity for participation by intended program beneficiaries in changing the institutions that the theorists felt to be at the root of delinquency and related troubles. Such theories were not well calculated to sell a program to either President Johnson or the Congress, however, and the "maximum feasible participation" phrase more or less slipped past those who most certainly would have weakened it had they understood this interpretation.

The use of the common-interest/partial-interest model suggests that the initiation of "maximum feasible participation" was based on the social theorists' contentions about where the public interest lay, rather than, for example, on the theorists' attempts to increase their own power. Paradoxically, however, this public-interest interpretation implied an attempt to restructure institutions by strengthening the capabilities of the beneficiaries of the poverty program to act in their own partial interest, thereby exacting better bargains from the rest of the citizenry. The institutions were created using federal money, the confrontations of the partial interests of the poor with the partial interests of the other parts of the community took place, and institutions were changed, in many cases in ways favorable to the poor.

Once the poverty institutions were created, they acted by and large in their own self-interests; it was this recourse to power bargaining that produced the favorable effects of the poverty program. The "maximum feasible participation" language backed by federal poverty funds created two kinds of institutions: those of the poor in the ghettos, and those of the bureaucrats in the poverty office and, ultimately, in the ghetto, too. These two interests maintained the program although it created, in a dialectic mode, even more powerful countervailing institutions. The larger communities confronted by the poor did not turn the other cheek; they exerted the power of their own interests, both locally and through the Congress, which passed legislation limiting and controlling the self-interest power of the poor. Using the power both of local officials and of the frightened middle class in the communities and a common-interest argument that questioned the legitimacy of using public money to finance political action by private self-interest groups, the countervailing forces pushed through Congress measures giving much more control over local poverty programs to local elected officials.

In the final analysis, this set of policies, designed largely in accordance with theorists' views of the common interest but directed by a clash of interests, achieved at least part of the designers' objectives for a number of years. It made changes in the living conditions of the ghetto poor, and in many cases led to permanent restructuring of the situations of these communities. It also carried with it the seeds of the destruction of its own political effectiveness. However, as is sometimes the case, it created a permanent bureaucracy whose primary interest was in its own preservation. The new poverty bureaucracy exists, but now as an old bureaucracy.

FEDERAL AID TO ELEMENTARY AND SECONDARY EDUCATION

In contrast to the "maximum feasible participation" idea, the program of federal aid to elementary and secondary education, made law during the two-year heyday of President Johnson's Great Society, stemmed initially from powerful partial-interest pressures outside the federal government. The program was substantially shaped, however, by political exigencies arising from the peculiar constitutional structure and traditions of the United States.

Public elementary and secondary education in the United States has historically been controlled and financed locally, by local school districts operating under constraints set up by the states. As early as the 1950s, however, school districts and states, realizing that demands on the educational system were growing faster than the resources available locally to finance it, largely because of the post-World War II baby boom, began turning to the federal government for financial assistance.(3)

The two major constraints that have, in greater or lesser degree, affected all proposals for federal social programs since the 1950s are limits on large-scale spending and fears of federal controls over local programs. Proposals for federal aid to education were made even more difficult by two additional factors. One of these, a traditional issue of American history, was the problem of the separation of church and state. Elementary and secondary schools run by religious bodies, primarily Roman Catholic parochial schools, were, like the public schools, also experiencing the effects of the baby boom and also wanted federal aid; but long American tradition and, perhaps, the Constitution (depending on the interpretation) were strongly against state aid to schools having religious affiliations. The second complication arose from an even more fiercely debated historical issue. In 1954, the Supreme Court of the United States definitively and unanimously declared state-maintained segregation of public schools to be unconstitutional. For more than a decade after this decision, however, the Southern states, where segregation had been official and legal, and sometimes the Northern states, resisted the constitutional dictate.

   Both the church/state and segregation issues led to the
formation of blocking coalitions in the Congress which opposed
any federal aid to education. Other factions arose as well:
those who would not vote for a bill without provisions for aid
to religious schools or those who would not vote for a bill
without a desegregation clause or those who would not vote for
a bill with such a clause.

   The stalemate broke in 1965. This was due in part both
to a shift of potential forces over time and to the major
changes that came about with President Kennedy's assassina-
tion and President Johnson's sweeping electoral triumph over
Senator Goldwater in 1964. However, the legislation passed
(Title I of the Elementary and Secondary Education Act) was
quite different from what had been proposed for ten years.
The change that made all the difference was a shift in perspective. The proposed aid came to be viewed not as aid to
schools, which were either religious or secular, segregated or
desegregated, but rather as aid to children, who could be
assisted regardless of religious belief or race. The major
portion of the aid was directed, in accordance with the rest of
President Johnson's "War on Poverty," to poor children, who
were presumed to be educationally underprivileged. Although
the aid was channeled through states and localities, it went to
schools attended by children, regardless of whether or not the
schools were segregated or had religious affiliations.

   This device was designed primarily to resolve the clash of
partial interests whose failure to achieve a bargain had until
then prevented the allocation of any federal aid, but its design
for aid to poor children embodied a very strong view that
underprivileged children rather than financially strained school
districts were the proper beneficiaries of educational aid in the
common interest. And, in fact, this view of the common
interest has prevailed over the pressure of strong special
interests in the years that the law has been in existence.
Once the breakthrough was made, pressures arose to change
the aid concept back to the original one of general federal aid
to politically powerful local educational authorities. The
pressure was particularly strong after the issue of legal
separation was resolved in favor of desegregation throughout
the nation during the decade that followed the passage of the
law in 1965. Such pressures, however, never came close to
forcing substantial change in the focus from aid for poor
children to general aid for school districts.

   This outcome hardly represents a complete triumph of the
common interest, or one view of the common interest, over
partial interests. The passage of the initial legislation created
a massive federal bureaucracy allied with changing state and
local bureaucracies, all of which had self-interests in keeping
the law as it was. Also, the money distributed to states and
localities was never used purely for poor children. Further-

more, it is always difficult to estimate what portion of funds
designed for a given major purpose are substituted for other
funds that would have been used for that purpose otherwise,
but are freed by their replacement to be used for other
expenditures (for example, for middle-class students).
Nonetheless, it does seem clear that the combined political
device/public-interest concept that shaped Title I of the
Elementary and Secondary Act of 1965 has largely directed the
law in the way intended. Furthermore, evidence in recent
years provides at least a preliminary indication that it has
been improving education for poor children.

WELFARE REFORM

Reform of the United States public assistance system, dis-
tinguishing this needs-based aid from social-insurance systems
that purport to be based on earned credits rather than needs,
has been an idea that has always received more backing from
intellectuals designing schemes than from any special-interest
group, including program beneficiaries. Indeed, in 1968, after
several hundred economists listed their names in a newspaper
advertisement endorsing the Negative Income Tax version of
welfare reform, Senator William Proxmire stated that he was not
surprised that several hundred economists were in favor of the
program and that he doubted whether he could find several
hundred of anyone else.

Although during the last half of the 1960s rapidly
growing public assistance costs and numbers of beneficiaries
led to some demands for change, taxpayers in general were not
then a well-defined special-interest group. These calls for
action merged with those on behalf of assistance recipients who
were hurt by a badly structured system into a general
public-interest-motivated debate over what should be done.
The major thrust was made by a group of economists, largely
within government, who carefully examined existing welfare
systems and designed the negative income tax proposal for a
new system intended to correct the perceived flaws of the
current ones.

The details of the negative income tax idea, initially
proposed in the late 1950s and early 1960s by conservative
economist Milton Friedman and liberal economist Robert
Lampman, are not crucial here. It attempted to turn fifty
state systems into one national system and to base eligibility
for benefits on need alone rather than on demographic category. In particular, it sought to bring in poor families in
which the father was present, as well as the mother-only
families who formed the vast majority of those covered under
the existing Aid to Families with Dependent Children (AFDC)

program.   By making coverage more general, it hoped to
eliminate the incentive perceived by the economists (although
perhaps not by the beneficiaries) for families to gain eligibility
by getting the father out of the house.   Indeed, incentives
formed the basis for the identifying characteristics of the
scheme, particularly incentives (also presumed by economists)
to induce assistance recipients to get onto the job rolls by
allowing them to earn wages without losing an equal amount of
assistance benefits.

The proposals were never taken seriously by politicians
during the Johnson Administration, who felt that they were too
radical, too gimmicky, and had no special-interest constituency
behind them.   When Nixon took office in 1969, the prediction
of sophisticated students of public policy was that the proposals never would be taken seriously except by economists.
In early 1969, however, Daniel Moynihan suggested to the
President both the public-interest importance of welfare reform
and the possible political benefits that might accrue from
reorganizing a system widely perceived to be in disarray.   The
plan that the Nixon administration developed was very much
like a modified negative income tax, and in the fall of 1969,
the President sent it to the Congress.   Largely on the basis of
public-interest arguments, it passed the House Ways and Means
Committee under the sponsorship of Chairman Wilbur Mills and
was ultimately passed by the House of Representatives.

In the Senate, however, the lack of any real special-
interest backing began to be apparent.   Combined with certain
design flaws (which could, perhaps, have been corrected),
this lack of political clout hurt the proposal badly.   In particular, the one constituency (albeit a very weak one) that
might have pushed for reform, welfare beneficiaries themselves, opposed it.   Their argument was that it was not
enough, and, indeed, the proposed conversion to a national
scheme provided little or nothing new for recipients in those
states that had already been paying relatively good benefits.
Many program advocates were shocked at the opposition of the
beneficiaries, but they should not have been so surprised that
the organized groups representing beneficiaries were concerned
with the effects of the proposal on their members, who were
already receiving benefits.   The real, new benefits would have
gone to those not then on the benefit rolls and not represented by these groups; and they carried even less political
weight.   The proposal never passed the Senate, and after one
more try, it disappeared.

What did happen, however, a few years later, was the
passage of a very similar program that applied only to the
aged and disabled category of assistance recipients.   The aged
and disabled led much less complicated lives than the people in
the other large category, Aid to Families with Dependent
Children, and were considered by the Congress to be much

more "deserving." In addition, the whole technically difficult question of work incentives was much less crucial for them. Perhaps overriding all this was that the aged did represent an identifiable and very powerful special interest.

In 1977-1978, President Carter nearly repeated Nixon's experience, except that Carter's plan did not even pass the House of Representatives. Generated again by public interest-based arguments about the needs of assistance beneficiaries and the needs of taxpayers in the states and localities which paid for half the public assistance, the Carter plan was devised by government economists and others, in wide consultation with holders of a variety of views. It, again, was based on negative income tax concepts, with the major addition of an extremely complex series of incentives and programs for jobs for the poor. Even though constrained by the Administration's budgetary imperatives, it was still quite costly, with the precise costs being in substantial dispute. Again, however, it lacked a constituency, and again it failed to pass. The one portion that did, in fact, have substantial special-interest backing, relief for states and localities, did continue to show some political promise.

Perhaps more strongly than any of the other examples, the experience of welfare shows the great difficulty of carrying through a major public policy based upon the public interest or, at least, the policy intellectual's interpretation of the public interest, alone. This is the kind of example that leads some analysts and policy makers in the United States to the conclusion that the public interest and policy analysis in the public interest do not count at all. The other examples here demonstrate otherwise, but certainly it is true that Senator Proxmire's several hundred economists by themselves carry little weight.

ENERGY LEGISLATION

That the United States was likely to run into supply problems of fossil fuels as domestic production dropped and dependence on petroleum imports increased was known to a few experts as early as the late 1960s. It first came to the attention of the public, however, in the summer of 1973, when regional short-ages in a few areas led to difficulties in obtaining gasoline. A few months later, this was followed by the much more massive effects of the Arab oil embargo and then the OPEC increase in petroleum prices. By the summer of 1974, however, the most difficult times had passed, and while the public was well aware of the shortage (although more than half believed the shortage was artificial, the result of a conspiracy by the big oil com-panies or others), nothing much was done about it.

When he assumed office in 1977, President Carter perceived a very strong national interest in reducing United
States dependence upon imported oil. Based on this common
interest, putative Energy Secretary James Schlesinger led a
group of other economists in the design of a new energy policy
which was to be embodied in new legislation. For two related
reasons, the policy was based very largely on decreasing the
demand for the scarce fuels, petroleum and natural gas, below
what it otherwise would have been by 1985, rather than increasing the domestic supply of petroleum and natural gas as
an alternative to imports. First, the administration's analysts
did not believe that the petroleum and natural gas could be
obtained from within American territory, except perhaps at a
truly exorbitant cost for supplies previously thought too
difficult to extract. Second, they felt that the economic
mechanisms that might have obtained these difficult supplies
and might have induced further exploration to find large new
reserves (which they did not think existed anyway) would give
vast "windfall profits" to the big oil companies, which they
wanted to avoid.

To achieve the desired savings of petroleum and natural
gas, therefore, the Administration came forth with a proposed
program substituting a series of market incentives for existing
price controls on petroleum and natural gas both to induce
additional energy conservation and to substitute coal, which
was in vast supply in the United States, for scarcer petroleum
and natural gas. A variety of taxes, subsidies, and related
devices were all devised to induce conservation and coal
substitution by raising oil and gas prices. The taxes were
designed to recapture the revenues from the increased prices
for the public rather than allowing private price increases to
give them to the oil companies. In many ways, this system
looked more workable than one that set up a large bureaucracy
to enforce rules and regulations designed to conserve and to
shift to coal.

What the designers failed to cope with was the fact that
sophisticated market devices of this nature are understandable
to economists, but not necessarily to anyone else (again, the
flaw exemplified by the negative income tax). In particular
they were difficult for lawyers, who think much more in terms
of rules, regulations, and enforcement, and who are in a
majority in the Congress.

Much more important, however, was that the designers of
the Administration's plan completely ignored the fact that the
plan was seen as hurting or helping many special interests.
Unsurprisingly, these special interests reacted in their own
interest, with the result verging on chaos. American
energy-producing interests had seen the President's proposals
both as substantially underplaying the possibilities of increasing the domestic supply of petroleum and natural gas and as

removing their chance of gaining the substantial profits they
would have obtained under less constrained workings of the
market system. Instead of substituting taxes for regulation of
the prices of oil and natural gas, they wanted the whole thing
freed so that prices could find their market level with the
resultant balancing of supply and demand. These energy-
producing interests, operating primarily through the Senators
and Representatives in the United States Congress from
Louisiana, Texas, and the states to the west, are extremely
powerful; and they had the power to disrupt the Administration's proposals completely.

At about the same time, with only a slight lag, liberal
and consumer groups saw the price increases that were intended, the movement toward deregulation, and the pressure
for further steps in this direction by the oil and gas interests, all as parts of a giant theft by the producers. Liberal
and consumer-interests groups are rather broader in scope
than the partial interests discussed above, such as the
poverty bureaucracy, state- and local-education interests,
welfare recipients, and oil and gas interests, and they are less
intense. In many cases, such broad but less focused interests
do not operate as effectively as the narrower ones. However,
this time they did, in part because of the fears induced by
general inflation and the common belief in an oil/gas conspiracy. Even so, these broader interests have probably been
less effective than the narrower ones. The point here is that
the President's public-interest-based proposal had little special
backing of its own, and it soon was ground between the
millstones of the various competing partial interests. The
debate shifted from the general-public interest to who was to
get what and who was to be boss. Little remained of any
general-interest considerations, except for an occasional weak
cry that unless the Congress did something to cut down on
imports, world markets would continue to drive the value of
the dollar down.

The authors of the proposal, who were excellent analysts
of the public interest which might result from the economic
efficiency of the marketplace, had forgotten that in the United
States economic issues put into the political arena tend to
become debates over the distribution of income and power.
Common-interest considerations acting through or allied with
partial interests have a fighting chance; the disembodied and
abstract common interest does not.

Thus, the common interest, particularly the common
interest as interpreted through the rationality of policy
analysis, is politically weak. There are probably examples in
wartime of common national interest considerations being so
predominant that events are swept before them regardless of
partial interests. In the United States, this may have been
the case for a full week or ten days after the Japanese attack
on Pearl Harbor, but probably not much longer.

All this has been obvious to many analysts in the process of public-policy making in the United States. They decried the lack of sophistication in the various attempts throughout the 1960s and 1970s to increase the rationality of the policy-making process by introducing more policy analysis. In many cases, the advocates of pure reform through policy analysis were not straw men, but they deserved the doubts of the skeptics. The cynics and skeptics talked about the triangle of outside interests, inside bureaucracies, and Congressional committees; and they wrote of government by mutual adjustment and bargaining between partial interests.

The trouble is, however, they too went too far. "Participation of the poor" was initiated out of a perception of the public interest. The history of federal aid to elementary and secondary education provides an example of major shaping of policy by a public-interest concept which was used to manipulate and reconcile partial interests. Even in the failed cases of welfare reform and energy policy, public-interest-shaping policy analysis would be necessary toward national goals. Bargaining among the partial interests would be likely to move further from the common interest than would unchanged policy.

What is needed is a new public-policy analysis that does not abandon the concept of rational achievement of the common interest, yet incorporates into its concept of rationality the idea that a policy so pure and untainted by partial interests is, in the final analysis, not rational at all because it becomes legislatively irrelevant. Such policy analysis will necessarily vary in different nations because of the differing institutions of pluralism. What is common to all, however, is the notion that these institutions and their effects must form a key part of the analysis.

NOTES

(1) Richard E. Flathman, The Public Interest (New York: Wiley, 1966), p. 25.
(2) Daniel P. Moynihan, Maximum Feasible Understanding (New York: The Free Press, 1969); see also Robert Levine, The Poor Ye Need Not Have With You: Lessons from the War on Poverty (Cambridge: MIT Press, 1970).
(3) Much of this legislative history of federal assistance to elementary and secondary education is taken from James L. Sundquist, Politics and Policy (Washington, D.C.: The Brookings Institution, 1968), Chapter V.
(4) Policy analysis definably stresses the common interest as a mode of argument. Policy analysts can be viewed most frequently as speaking for their views of the common

interest, simply because the power of their own partial
interests is so meagre as to not be worth bargaining
with.   Recently, they have been forming self-interest
lobbies, however.

2 Citizens' Action Groups in the German Political System*
Uwe Thaysen and Stephen Artner

A lively debate presently centers around the role of Burger-initiativen (citizens' action groups, literally "citizens' initiatives") in the West German political system. The influence of citizens' action groups has been established beyond all doubt in recent years. The nature of this influence, however, remains in dispute. The Bundesverband Burgerinitiativen Umweltschutz (BBU: Federal Association of Citizens' Action Groups for Environmental Protection), the largest umbrella organization of Burgerinitiativen in the Federal Republic, can claim to have become a "leading, at times predominant force in questions of the future."(1)   Critics, on the other hand, regard such groups less as vanguards of the future than as "bludgeons against progress" which strive to repeal the Enlightenment through anarchy and "volumeocracy" - the rule not of the majority, but of the loudest.(2)   The Schmidt government has not stilled the debate over citizens' action groups: in response to parliamentary interpellation, it has welcomed their basically constructive attitude but called for further attention to their (largely unspecified) "problematics."(3)

The uncertainty surrounding citizens' action groups stems not least from their diversity. No generally accepted definition embracing all such groups has yet been developed. This discussion will therefore examine a few general hypotheses

---

*This contribution is based on a report that Uwe Thaysen wrote for a Symposium of the Parliamentary Assembly of the Council of Europe held in Strasbourg, March 30-31, 1978. The Symposium dealt with "The Role of Political Parties in the Development of Parliamentary Democracy."

concerning Burgerinitiativen which can contribute to such a
definition. In addition, it will address the decisive practical
question of the political system's possible reactions to this
phenomenon. To evaluate the Burgerinitiativen themselves and
to suggest their probable consequences are thus the objectives
of this interim assessment.

DEVELOPMENT AND SCOPE OF CITIZENS' ACTION

Historically, citizens' action movements are not a novel development. "Citizens' action," in the broadest sense, has
propelled a broad range of social transformation in numerous
countries over a span of centuries. At least since the French
Revolution, in its origins a bourgeois rebellion, popular
initiative has been among the fundamental values of western
democracies.
        In the thirty-year history of the Federal Republic of
Germany, however, the rise of citizens' action groups since
the late 1960s indeed represents a new departure. Their
introduction and growth, as John Elliot notes, have marked a
change from general passivity to a new activism in West
German popular political participation.(4) According to some
accounts, their total membership rivals or even exceeds that of
the established political parties. The assistant chairman of the
BBU has speculated that his group, were it to compete in
elections as a political party, would attract more votes than
the liberal FDP.(5) In 1973 the Office of the Federal
President estimated the total membership of Burgerinitiativen at
1.5 million, only 200,000 less than that of all the political
parties combined.(6) Of course, difficulties in defining both
Burgerinitiativen themselves and the criteria of membership in
them make precise figures impossible to obtain. Public opinion
polls, however, confirm substantial sympathy and active
support for citizens' action groups throughout the past
decade.(7)
        In identifying the causes of this phenomenon, one must
distinguish between the fundamental structural factors which
called the citizens' action movement into being, and the specific, as it were, "accidental" factors which have conditioned
its development in West Germany during the past ten or twelve
years.
        The Federal Republic of Germany, like other western
democracies, has witnessed the transformation of the classical
liberal minimal state into a pluralistic welfare state catering to
the wide-ranging social needs of its citizens. This transformation is the primary structural determinant of West
Germany's citizens' action movements. For, while the citizen
gains greater security and creative scope from the welfare

state, he or she also becomes increasingly dependent upon its largesse. When the various levels of government fail to provide services, or provide them inadequately, the citizen is virtually forced to take political action. In a pluralistic society, this action must be collective: effective influence requires unions, interest groups, political parties, and, increasingly, citizens' action groups.

A subtle difference in objectives, however, distinguishes the Burgerinitiativen from political parties and traditional interest groups. The latter have generally protested a lack of services and demanded additional government interventions, thus promoting the emergence and growth of the modern welfare state. Burgerinitiativen, in contrast, characteristically react against what are perceived as excesses of the modern state, calling for the prevention or correction of mistaken or misdirected governmental activities.

Legislatures are quite limited in their ability to restrain the modern state, whose growing authority results largely, if often indirectly, from their own enactments. Parties, as heterogeneous, integrative forces, usually limit their pronouncements to generalities and avoid entanglement in the specifics of governmental and administrative interventions. Nor does the law serve primarily to protect the individual from the state. Thus, as governmental intervention increasingly characterizes every area of modern life, a "representation gap" prevents citizens from countering this intervention through judicial and elective institutions. Along with these "primary organizations," Burgerinitiativen have therefore arisen as "secondary organizations," not as "early warning systems," as some have contended, but more accurately as "too-late warning systems," as correctives of the interventions of government and the insufficient responsiveness of parliaments, parties, and courts.(8)

If the representation gap inherent in the modern welfare state is the essential structural determinant of the citizens' action groups, a series of circumstances and events has conditioned their development in West Germany during the past several years. A few of these conditional determinants are:
° 	a reduction in economic growth first encountered during the recession of 1966-67, and growing concomitant conflicts over the distribution of wealth;
° 	continuing high demand for state services, further increased by the reform policy of the SPD-FDP government after 1969;
° 	political sensitization through the student rebellions and extra-parliamentary opposition during the years 1967-1970;
° 	the challenge of the Brandt government in 1969 to "risk more democracy";
° 	the designation of 1970 as the Year of Environmental Protection in Europe;

- a general questioning and reevaluation of traditional norms;
- the oil crisis of 1973-74 and subsequent efforts to maintain West Germany's economic standing, particularly national energy policies with their inevitable consequences upon employment and the environment;
- growing popular disenchantment with government and political parties following the parliamentary elections of 1976.

Such trends and circumstances have supplied the specific context in which Burgerinitiativen have begun to operate in response to their fundamental cause, the representational deficits of the modern state.

CONSTITUTIONALITY

Burgerinitiativen largely bypass legislatures and political parties, addressing themselves directly to the principal executors of the policies of the modern welfare state, the administrative bureaucracy. Traditionally, legislative bodies could either arrive at, or simply assume, a consensus as to the proper degree of state involvement in the social and economic spheres. Bureaucracies carried out the clear-cut and politically neutral task of implementing that consensus. To the extent that legislatures and parties now fail to specify the details of state activity, bureaucracies are enabled, and indeed compelled, actively to shape social policy. As citizens become aware of this, they turn directly to administrative organs, not only to protest measures already taken, but to demand particular actions in advance. Only when such appeals fail do they have recourse to parties, legislatures, and public opinion. Citizens' action groups now come to rival the political parties, not merely reacting after the fact as secondary organizations, but demanding from the primary organizations the right to equal participation in determining policy objectives.

Frequently, only open conflict between Burgerinitiativen and administrative organs will stimulate elected bodies to take notice of popular grievances and react. When parties and legislatures then devise feasible political solutions, Burgerinitiativen have succeeded in bridging the representation gap of the modern state. Reminding parliament, government, and bureaucracy of their proper respective positions within a system of divided powers, they not only protect individual rights, but also provide a kind of safeguard for the constitution. Functioning in this manner, citizens' action groups undoubtedly conform to the West German Basic Law, the constitution of the Federal Republic, and indeed help to implement

the democratic ideals it represents. Hence there can be no
doubt that Burgerinitiativen are compatible in principle with
the constitution.

Of course, relations between citizens' groups and governmental bodies are not always so remarkably free of tension.
Parties and legislatures often react unclearly or not at all;
they may also make decisions opposed by Burgerinitiativen.
The latter then sometimes deduce a right to resistance or even
to violence in promoting the popular will. The theorectical
discussion of Burgerinitiativen must therefore be supplemented
with an empirical examination of them and their place in
German political life.

POLITICAL APPRAISAL

While Burgerinitiativen differ significantly in objectives,
methods, and scope, they tend to exhibit a number of common
characteristics. Burgerinitiativen typically demand expanded
opportunities for political participation. They push for change
in the official decision-making structures. In this respect
they differ fundamentally from traditional interest groups,
which accept and operate within the existing institutional
framework. While interest groups unquestioningly support the
representative system within which their particular concerns
can be effectively addressed, citizens' action groups hope to
modify the antiplebiscitary Basic Law in the direction of more
direct democracy and less harmonization of differing or
conflicting interests.

The border line between Burgerinitiativen and traditional
interest groups is fluid, but may be defined by the objectives
both groups claim to pursue. Burgerinitiativen claim to
struggle, not for special interests, but for those of the
community at large. Their demand for greater participation
rests upon their putative unbiased perception of the common
good. Even when frustrated interest groups transform themselves into Burgerinitiativen for transparently tactical reasons,
they confront governmental bodies with far greater claims to
legitimacy than before. In presenting their case, interest
groups must accept the burden of proof that their objectives
are consistent with the common good. Citizens' action groups,
on the other hand, simply assume that they embody the public
interest, and challenge opponents to prove the contrary.
Such a presumption, needless to say, cannot be recognized
a priori in a pluralistic democracy.

As a rule, citizens' action groups are thematically,
temporally, and geographically limited. "Horizontal consolidation," the cooperation of Burgerinitiativen from the local
through the international level, has largely been confined to

those in the environmental field. Typically formed to address a specific issue or grievance, Burgerinitiativen are likely to dissolve once their particular demands have been met, hence the lament of successful groups, "another victory, and we are lost."

This limitation of citizens' action groups underscores their dissimilarity to political parties, which must appeal to varying interests on a large number of issues. If citizens' groups were to compete with the parties, they would need to broaden their programs and popular following. "Green lists" campaigning almost exclusively on environmental concerns have proved unable to mount a significant challenge to the parties in Land (provincial) elections during the past two years.

Burgerinitiativen encourage membership, but not at the expense of organization. Indeed, as they grow older they often attain a degree of organization comparable to that of the established interest groups. Financial and legal considerations are among the most important reasons for this development. Constituted as an eingetragener Verein (registered nonprofit organization), a citizens' group can gain the financial support and legal standing to take part in administrative and judicial proceedings. Strategically, it continues to operate as a Burgerinitiative.

A study by Barbara Borsdorf-Ruhl discovered that only half the Burgerinitiativen allow anyone to become a member, and that most have an active membership ranging from only twenty to thirty. Fully 57 percent of the groups questioned had enacted official statutes.(9) Thus, citizens' action groups are hardly the amorphous bodies their critics sometimes charge them of being. They may encourage membership, but they are by no means disorganized.

A common mistake is to judge the goals pursued by Burgerinitiativen solely in light of their social composition. Although predominantly middle class in membership, citizens' action groups are not bound to the pursuit of narrow class interests. They have been largely unable to activate those elements of society that are underrepresented for various reasons in all other political organizations at all levels. Nonetheless, their achievements frequently benefit others beyond their own membership. The advantages of recreational parks or depolluted rivers, for example, can hardly be confined to an exclusive circle, and are often most directly appreciated by the least privileged classes of society.

This is not to suggest that citizens' action groups invariably and consciously pursue altruistic or philanthropic aims, but only that they can serve a general, "inclusive interest"(10) even when motivated by the desire to increase their members' own material advantage. Referring to proecology initiatives, Mayer-Tasch goes so far as to claim that "the citizens' groups' successes in this field benefit the lower

classes of the population to a greater extent than the so-
called privileged."(11) Even a less optimistic view would
suggest that society as a whole can reap dividends from
Burgerinitiativen despite their frequently restricted social
composition.

Since the appearance of Claus Offe's essay "Burgerinitiativen und Reproduktion der Arbeitskraft im Spatkapi-
talismus" (Citizens' Action Groups and the Reproduction of
Labor Power in Late Capitalism),(12) a common criticism of
citizens' action groups has contended that they arise within
and relate exclusively to the productive sector of the economy.
Analyzed in class terms, they can, therefore, never be progressive. However, the facts have confuted this charge, for
environmental protection has become a leading concern of
Burgerinitiativen. Following the oil crisis of 1973 and subsequent shortages of energy, ecology-oriented citizens'
initiatives have increasingly affected the productive sector.
They positively and negatively influence employment through
the bearing they have upon hundreds of thousands of jobs.
The Schmidt government more or less directly accuses Burgerinitiativen of reducing West Germany's rate of economic growth
by 1 percent by tying up 25 billion DM in administrative and
judicial proceedings.(13) However such arguments may be
assessed in particular, the direct effects of Burgerinitiativen
in and upon the productive sector should force governments at
all levels to include them in their political and legislative cal-
culations.

Distrust of citizens' action groups has fed upon the
theoretical and actual willingness of some to break the law, to
combine a strategy of negotiation with calculated acts of
violence.(14) Such an attitude toward the law has frequently
given citizens' groups in general a reputation as subversive
revolutionary movements. The words and some of the deeds of
certain student groups in particular suggest either that their
propaganda cannot be taken seriously, or that the suspicions
they arouse are not without foundation.

Theories of "state interventionism" and "state monopoly
capitalism" regard local and national authorities as the instruments of a ruling economic class. Student proponents of
illegal action urge the establishment of "counterpowers" that
are meant not only to break, but in the long run to destroy,
existing law. Citizens' action groups, as well as legislatures
and "bourgeois" parties, are viewed in Leninist terms as strategic forums for mass activity. Even without such an ideological basis, the previously mentioned certainty of knowing the
common good cannot infrequently inspire fanaticism. Further,
the bewildering complexity and the resulting emotional over-
tones of many current issues can lead to violent outbursts only
tenuously connected with ideology.

Those willing to engage in violence characteristically refuse to let themselves be questioned - least of all by the "bourgeoisie." Their subjective certainty of the truth permits no inquiry. Otherwise, they would at least wonder whether their actions do not provoke the very police state whose emergency they claim to fear. From a Marxist point of view, some would also have to ask themselves, as did Georg Lukacs (Legalitat und Illegalitat, 1920), whether their "romantics of violence" are not in the end a kowtow before the bourgeois state, a kowtow which magnifies that state in the consciousness not only of the bourgeoisie, but of the revolutionaries themselves.

The avoidance of violence is not only a problem for the state, but a challenge to the citizens' action groups themselves. As a rule, these groups want nothing to do with violence. Many are cooperating with one another in identifying and handling radical, violence-prone minorities. At large antinuclear demonstrations, they have been instrumental in preventing clashes between communistic groups and the police.

Their concern for protest and change has misled a few citizens' action groups into forgetting the democratic necessity of clearly established procedures and institutions. The overwhelming majority, however, unreservedly adhere to legal and nonviolent patterns of action.

In summary, one may conclude that citizens' action groups represent no threat to the West German Basic Law. Rather, they are a complement to the parties and legislatures which can even point out to them their proper constitutional positions. Burgerinitiativen must be firmly defended against their detractors, both those who view them simply as the harbingers of anarchy and those who would use them as instruments in the class struggle.

As long as parties and parliaments fulfill their representational responsibilities, Burgerinitiativen are necessarily limited in subject matter, life span, and scope. Their organizational structure is solid enough, and their programs and following wide enough, to make consultation or cooperation with federal and municipal authorities a distinct possibility. Burgerinitiativen should not be condemned because of the violence perpetrated by a small minority.

How can and should the state behave in regard to citizens' action groups? The answer depends on the future development of the groups, which can be predicted in part on the basis of the liberal state's transformation, however incomplete, into the pluralistic welfare state of today. This transformation increasingly forces the citizen to take organized collective action. In addition, recently established opportunities for greater political participation (e.g., in municipal charters, federal construction, city planning, and administrative procedures) create permanent legal claims.

Resulting judicial victories have encouraged the formation of more citizens' groups. After a phase of sober assessment and perhaps some retrenchment, Burgerinitiativen will cease to be sociopolitical novelties and will become an accepted feature of pluralistic democracy.

Some evidence suggests that because of the behavior of government, unions, and parties, and because of their own use of violence, the national proecology Burgerinitiativen passed their zenith in the spring of 1977. Nonetheless, they remain a potential threat to the established parties. This threat, however, is no cause for alarm about the parliamentary system of government as a whole. State institutions, particularly the legislatures, are not in danger. To the extent that citizens' action groups become serious competitors with the parties, they will need to become broadly based, integrative electoral movements, thereby (as long as they strictly observe the Basic Law) simply replacing the parties that have failed. Burgerinitiativen are thus a threat only to ineffective political parties. The remoteness of this threat is illustrated by the serious disagreements among the ecological Burgerinitiativen themselves over issues such as the Radicals Decree and the use of artificial fertilizer in the Third World.

Representation of citizens' everyday interests through Burgerinitiativen will in all probability increase. Burgerinitiaven could conceivably endanger the existing political parties, but only by developing into new parties in the presence of which parliamentary government could still continue.

Finally, possible reactions to Burgerinitiativen can be indicated only briefly. To assure their own survival, the political parties will have to concern themselves increasingly with the issues addressed by the major national citizens' action groups. Because of the well-known "localization of politics," municipal authorities and, to a lesser extent, provincial and federal governments will have to cope with an avalanche of demands for greater participation. Municipal charters should, therefore, be broadened to include the whole range of participatory, and especially consultative, rights: public grievance, petition, and referendum; participation in city council committees, advisory boards, community work and legal planning; public forums, hearings, question periods, and assemblies; greater access to official documents, etc.

At the local level, certain elective institutions are indeed in danger, namely the Gemeinderate (municipal councils). Their prerogatives must be safeguarded against citizens' groups, which can only constitute "initiatives from the people addressed to the people." Legislatures, the people's central representative organs, must retain the last word at all levels. Thus, the municipal councils should be strengthened, particularly against a highly traditional form of coziness between Burgerinitiativen and administrative officials.

The municipal councils face the same problem as do Burgerinitiativen: The growing complexity of the modern federal state renders the proper locus of effective participation increasingly difficult to determine. A complete disentanglement of federal, provincial, and local responsibilities has become impossible. Thus, to counter the growing constraints on local autonomy, municipal councils should be granted a greater voice in supraregional and national decisions. The activities of local Burgerinitiativen can be effective only when municipal authorities receive either greater scope to make their own decisions or a greater role alongside Parliament in shaping national policy.

Although they present no real danger to the parties and legislatures, citizens' action groups do threaten to block innovations and, through ever-greater participatory rights and use of litigation, to bring the entire political system to a halt. Failure to define clearly and to harmonize the areas, objects, and loci of participation within a federal system can only accelerate this trend. And, in addition to these political and constitutional considerations, the economic significance of Burgerinitiativen necessitates a clearer definition of their functions and limitations in a pluralistic federal state.

To the extent that parties and parliaments fail to provide convincing answers and clear decisions, courts must step in, and Burgerinitiativen become a danger to the political parties, though not yet to the legislatures. This applies particularly to the rational legal structuring of participatory rights. To the extent that parties and elected bodies fail to offer citizens of the pluralistic welfare state meaningful opportunities for political participation, they cut the citizens and themselves off from chances to learn.

Such a development does not help to resolve the constant paradox of democracy, which must ever bring forth the mature, informed citizen it theoretically assumes in advance. Citizens' action groups, along with parties and parliaments, can contribute to this educational process. The parliamentary system's characteristic ability to learn, and its resulting social tranquility, are at stake. Optimal conditions of cooperation between Burgerinitiativen and the state are thus not the end, but the prerequisite, of political enlightenment.

NOTES

(1)   Hans-Helmuth Wustenhagen, chairman of the BBU until autumn 1977, quoted in "Burgerinitiativen - Mehr Stimmen als die F.D.P.," Wirtschaftswoche, vol. 31, no. 16, April 7, 1977.

(2)   Hans-Jochen Vogel, "Wenn Burger was wollen. Auch
       Burgerinitiativen Haben ihre Grenzen," Die Zeit, June 9,
       1972; Herbert Kremp, "An diesen Parteien vorbie. Die
       Burgerinitiative: Reaktion   auf   die   Versteinerte
       Demokratie?," Die Welt, February 18, 1977.
(3)   BT-Drs 8/24 of March 3, 1977.
(4)   John D. Elliot, "The Changing Style of Political
       Participation in West Germany." Paper delivered at the
       1977 annual meeting of the American Political Science
       Association, September 1-4, 1977.
(5)   Hans Gunter Schumacher, quoted in Wirtschaftswoche,
       op. cit., p. 8.
(6)   Bulletin des Presse- und Informationsamtes der
       Bundesrefierung, no. 15, p. 125, February 13, 1973.
(7)   See, for example, the Infas public-opinion poll of April-
       May, 1973.
(8)   For the terminology see Heinz Grossman's epilogue to his
       collection Burgerinitiative: Schritte zur Veranderung?,
       Frankfurt am Main, 1971, p. 169.
(9)   Barbara Borsdorf-Ruhl, Burgerinitiativen im Ruhrgebiet,
       Essen, 1973.
(10)   The term derives from Eckart Pankoke, "Politische
       Partizipation und Liberale Demokratie," Liberal, vol. 14
       (1972), p. 357.
(11)   Peter Cornelius Mayer-Tasch, Die Burgerinitiativen-
       bewegung. Der Aktive Burger als Rechts- und Politik-
       wissenschaftliches Problem. Hamburg, 1976, 9. 93.
(12)   In Heinz Grossman (ed.), op. cit.
(13)   Cf. Klaus Altman's interview on the television program
       "Bericht aus Bonn" with the broadcast on September 23,
       1977 with parliamentary state secretary in the Economics
       Ministry, Martin Gruner.
(14)   Offe, in Grossman, op. cit.

II
Energy Policy

3 Citizens' Participation in Decision-Making Processes in Energy and Environmental Policy

Horst Zillessen

THE NECESSITY OF CITIZENS' PARTICIPATION

The rise in the <u>Burgerinitiative</u> movement in the Federal Republic has led some West Germans to doubt whether the present form of representative democracy is capable of dealing effectively with the broad range of demands directed at it. The development of the representative system does not appear to guarantee that the democratic fundamentals of individual freedom and political self-determination can be maintained intact.

This system presumes that constitutionally devised organs, to which the people have transferred their "power," undertake legally authorized functions of sovereignty so that they can impartially balance all relevant factors of influence in the service of the common interest. The system is, therefore, based on a number of presuppositions. There are structural presuppositions about the conditions for decision making, and there are subjective presuppositions about the decision makers. In the reality of an industrial society these presuppositions are less and less likely to be found. <u>Burgerinitiativen</u> are not merely symptoms of a temporary failure of the political parties; they are also indicators of the need for a higher general level of citizen participation as a necessary corrective to a predominantly representative system.

The large number of <u>Burgerinitiativen</u> in the area of environmental protection indicates that the representative system is no longer sufficient to realize a common interest, which overlaps individual interests, and that the equality of the people and their influence on policy can no longer be preserved. <u>Burgerinitiativen</u> today partially fill the gaps that representative democracy has produced.

FAILURE OF THE POLITICAL PARTIES

That many citizens today seek to exercise their political rights
of self-determination outside the political parties, outside the
sphere of representation, in the form of direct influence can
be attributed to structural weaknesses in the system of
representation. The political parties have also contributed to
this phenomenon, through both subjective failure and structural problems. At the October 1977 CDU Congress on
"Energy and Environment," Roman Herzog spoke of a "lack of
sensibility by the parties concerning new problems and new
states of awareness of the population."(1) The complaint is
becoming louder everywhere that the parties have lost the
essential nearness to the people, and that what is repeatedly
discussed under the catch word Staatsverdrossenheit (governmental intractability) is in reality a Parteiverdrossenheit
(party intractability). It obviously results from the division
between the hypothetical will of the people and the empirical
will of the people that has become problematic. Hence, an
increasingly intolerable political alienation of the people has
resulted.
     The close integration of the parties with the large
interest groups as well as with the administration strengthens
this trend. It leads to an interaction between leadership
groups that is regulated by the rules and provisions of the
Bundestag and the common leadership of the Federal ministries, which ends on the party level with a clear predominance
of the Apparat, the party apparat, and the party leadership.
If real influence on decisions is taken as a measure, representation of the public is limited to a relatively small leadership class from parties and interest groups.(2)
     Parties must often repress the determination and capa-
bility for action of particular interests as long as they do not
concern a recognized theme in the marketplace of political
opinions. But because the broadening range of public policy
forces the assertion of a continual stream of new interests, the
number of those interests which fall through the nets of this
system of problem management is likewise necessarily increased. The size of the parties causes intraparty integra-
tional problems. The parties, therefore, often succumb to the
danger of treating their own problems as political ones. They
must often occupy themselves more with internal problems than
with societal ones.
     The possibility of harmonizing all empirical interests
within one all-encompassing common interest is highly limited.
Frequently the independence and freedom of choice of the
representative are either restricted by party ties or links to
interest groups, or they are rendered insignificant by the
dominant influence of such organizations. An oversimplified

conclusion may thus be formulated: The will of the people is less improved upon by representatives than it is guided in a specific direction.

For a long time this development has not been perceived as being problematical.   In the meantime, the indices are growing - confirmed by Rudolf Wildenmann in his survery for Capital magazine - that the schism between parties and the electorate can have serious consequences.

Fears of this sort are confirmed not only by the rise of the Burgerinitiative movement.   Representative surveys on important societal problem areas also signal an alarmingly low level of citizens' confidence in politicians.   According to a "scale of confidence" devised by the Institute for Applied Social Sciences (Infas), the credibility of Burgerinitiativen and environmental organizations is almost twice as high as that of politicians on the subject of the environmental compatibility of industrial settlements and nuclear power plants.   Even if the credibility of Burgerinitiativen is compared with that of the more strongly normative entity, "the state," according to the Capital survey, only 34.7 percent of the population give their sympathy to the state, while 34.4 percent decide in favor of Burgerinitiativen and 31.9 percent prefer to judge according to the particular situation.   If one further notes that 35 percent of the population would welcome the admission of Burgerinitiativen to participate in elections, and that 25 percent can conceive of voting for a Burgerinitiative instead of a party, representative democracy is obviously in an alarming state. As Wildenmann says, "Even if the parties do not want to admit it, the loss of confidence is already greater than the Federal Republic can tolerate."(3)

LOCAL DECISION MAKING

Representative democracy's situation makes the demands for greater and improved possibilities for citizens' participation unavoidable.   The assumptions, provisions, and effects of decisions with such far-reaching consequences as those in the energy and environmental field must be adequately discussed; their consequences for the individual must be made clear. Moreover, if such decisions encroach upon the living habits of the population, as they do in city planning or energy con- servation, in the long run they will probably be carried out successfully only through intensive participation by citizens.

The desire for more effective forms of citizens' parti- cipation has already been partially met by legislators.   At least those citizens affected by a renovation plan can possibly exert infuence on the structural form of their environment.   The Town Planning Promotion Act provides for the following steps:

Step 1: A preliminary inquiry into "the necessity of the renovation, the social, structural and town planning conditions and relationships"§(4.1 Town Planning Promotion Act) and the detrimental consequences. At the same time there is to be a determination of the attitude and participational preparedness of the property owners, tenants, lessees, and others entitled to its use.

Step 2: A discussion of the community's ideas with those affected (§4.2), the results of which are to be contained in the report on the preliminary investigations.

Step 3: The community's decision on the formal determination of the area to be renovated is to be expressed as an ordinance that is to be given to the higher administrative authorities for approval. The proposal is attached to the report on the preliminary investigation. Public announcement is then made of both the ordinance and the approval by the administrative authorities (§5.1-3).

Step 4: Formation of a social plan that is to be continuously supplemented during the renovation by discussions with those directly affected. Other considerations taken into account are employment, business and familial conditions, age structure, living necessities, and social implications (§8.2).

Step 5: Discussions with those affected about the new form the area to be renovated is to take and about the possibility of their participation. If desired, an adequate period of time is to be allotted for comments to be prepared. A report is to be written on the discussions (§9).

The Town Planning Promotion Act undoubtedly represents a step in the right direction. Certainly the possibility cannot be excluded that the participational opportunities offered here are often, in fact, no more than participational embellishments of bureaucratic decisions. In such a case, not only a determined engagement by the parties would be necessary, but the farthest-reaching organizational, personal, and material support for those citizens who want to assert their participational rights would also be necessary. In a highly organized society, citizens' participation requires organizational support if it is to be more than a political declamation.

PLANNING CELLS

A new departure for participation by citizens in the area of city and environmental planning is offered by the "planning cells" proposed by Peter Dienel. A planning cell is a group of 25 lay planners who are randomly chosen, are allowed three weeks away from their work, and are reimbursed by the government. Together with two members of the relevant government department and two people who guide the proceedings, such a group seeks to develop feasible solutions to problems of valuation, supervision, or planning that are presented.(4) This form of participation is useful in cases in which no determination has been made of those who would be directly affected by a certain plan. An example of this might be the planning of a new section of a city. With the use of a planning cell, an attempt is made to bring into the decision-making process the widest variety of wishes and needs.

The advantages of this procedure are that participation by citizens is institutionalized and can be usefully incorporated into the administrative-planning process. Because of the random selection of cell members, all social groups have an equal chance to bring their opinions into the planning process. Practical experiences with planning cells have shown that all participants availed themselves of this chance to a surprisingly strong degree, regardless of social class. In this manner additional ideas and impulses could flow into the planning process, and the plans and actions of the administration could be better aligned with the actual wishes, needs, and interests of the population.

The concept of the planning cell assumes that local and higher courts will keep a register of those designs worthy of treatment. The appropriate parliamentary body decides which subject will be assigned to a planning cell, or it offers the cell a choice of a number of subjects. The group working as a planning cell should be manageable in size and have at its disposal both a constant staff and enough time to finish their task. An accidental bias in the composition of the group could be compensated for if more than one planning cell dealt with the same problem.

The planning cell offers chances to individual citizens to take a larger part in the concerns of the community and, thereby, also participate in its decisions.

ORGANIZING FOR PARTICIPATION

An improvement in participational possibilities in the environmental field must begin with granting the individual concrete opportunities to influence decisions. In addition, a structure for participation is needed under the given societal conditions that links ongoing and spontaneous forms of participation with one another so that participation is possible and useful in the preparation, execution, and supervision of political and administrative decisions. At the same time it should guarantee that attempts at participation are not threatened by lack of time and materials.

As a model for one such structure, an organization for local participation by citizens is suggested. It would provide for the discussion of all environmentally relevant questions and problems in a citizens' assembly. In larger cities, such a citizens' assembly could be formed within spatially delineated city districts, the borders of which could be established on the basis of historically or politically plausible criteria. For clarification of complicated technical questions, the citizens' assembly would employ a committee chosen from its ranks. With the help of specific technical advisory bodies and planning cells, the citizens' committee would then be in the position to clear up problems of detail and, if necessary, to answer public questions posed by the citizens' assembly after consultation with the appropriate administrative body. The citizens' assembly and the citizens' committee would be supported organizationally and personally, especially in their preparation for assemblies and sessions, by an independent citizens' bureau. Local Burgerinitiativen could also be engaged in this participational process; they would be supported by the citizens' bureau to the same extent as the other bodies and could become active in the citizens' assembly as well as attempting to exert direct influence on the city legislature and administration.

After such a participational process is completed, it is quite possible that a final citizens' assembly could advance concrete demands and develop firmly outlined aims. The more decisive the vote of the citizens' assembly and the larger the participation in the vote, the less the political representatives can disregard it. Thus, it would be clear to the participants that to take part in this participational process is worthwhile, and new prospects for intensive participation in the fashioning of the environment would thereby open up. The variety of procedures and methods that are included in this model further guarantee that the complexity of the environmental problem is adequately taken into account.

APPROVAL PROCEDURES FOR THE
FEDERAL EMISSIONS PROTECTION ACT

Article 4 of the Federal Emissions Protection Act provides for an approval procedure for the establishment and operation of plants which have detrimental effects on the environment. Article 4 also includes possibilities for participation by affected citizens. Of course, doubts have arisen in this case - as they have over the corresponding regulations in the Town Planning Promotion Act and the Federal Construction Act - about the effectiveness of these possibilities.

According to the procedures, the authorities ratifying the proposal should make it public in their official publications and in the daily newspapers. This public notice is usually made in a small-print announcement that is not prominent enough to make the procedure widely known. It is necessary to aim for preparation of a public discussion through a full explanation of the present controversies in the daily newspapers, accompanied and supplemented by public announcement of activities put on by the political parties.

The proposal and the attached documents should be displayed by the authorities so that third parties may judge whether and to what extent they could be affected by the plant. Of course, the examination of these documents is only permitted during regular office hours, which represents a considerable inconvenience, particularly if no copying facilities are made available. Only a summary can be mimeographed, but summaries seldom include the details upon which the approval depends.

To the degree that the authorities charged with approval consider it necessary, they seek the advice of experts. Whether this, however, takes into account the arguments of the affected citizens and answers their questions can be ascertained only in the discussion period, during which the objections of those affected are treated. If this is to be more than a process for the rejection of objections, it should be endowed with the trappings of a judicial proceeding. Its conduct should be prepared by the authorities in conjunction with not only the applicant, but also with representatives of those objecting. In that way the decision about which documents may be considered and which representatives of those objecting may be admitted is not left to the judgment of the assembly leader, who is named by the ratifying authorities. Finally, the discussion period should not treat the objections alone. The opinions of the applicants and of those objecting, as well as the point of view of the authorities, should be made the subject of the hearing.

THE WIEDENFELS MODEL

A concrete beginning for a problem-oriented approval procedure is offered by the Wiedenfels model, developed in 1973 at a conference of the Protestant Academy of Baden. It begins with this question: How should the scientific appraisal of the environmental consequences of the plant be regulated? The decisive point is that the judgment of technical-scientific questions is always tied to normative questions, for what are understood to be "considerable disadvantages and dangers" obviously are often differently assessed by plant managers, those affected, and the authorities. Therefore, in order to inform the affected citizen as comprehensively and objectively as possible, a public discussion of independently devised parallel opinions is suggested. The procedure would then begin with agreement among the participants on a list of questions and a timetable for the investigation process. The participants would be the applicant or applicants, the ratifying authorities, and those persons affected by the environmental impact who have organized themselves in the form of a Burgerinitiative.

        The list of questions should include all those that appear important to the participating groups; they should then be reviewed in a public hearing. Reference could be made to the application for approval, in which the applicant must, among other things, point out the expected environmental burdens. Each participating group would elect an advisor according to those aspects of the case that appear important to it. The advisor would be presented with the list of questions. In this manner a comparison of the opinions should be guaranteed. The applicant would bear the cost of the opinions.

        In private deliberations, the participants in the procedure would then work out a joint opinion from the three individual opinions, even if this led to diverging individual votes. This joint opinion, as well as the individual opinions, should be promptly made public so that the affected population can suf-ficiently inform themselves before the public hearing. At the hearing the representatives of the authorities and the applicant must express their opinions along with the advisors. A citi-zen's participation in the discussion should be made dependent on a written notification in order to facilitate the organization of the hearing. The intended result of this process is a rec-ommendation to the authorities responsible for approving the application, which would be certain to influence the final decision. Beyond this, or in place of a recommendation, the hearing could also lead to suggestions which, for example, call upon the legislature to change certain standards or procedures, upon the parties to examine economic or regional policies, or upon the academic world to develop new core areas of research. Finally, the aim of the approval procedure is to both publicly and rationally consider the pros and cons associated with the planned structure and to make sure that the decision is subject to general agreement.

        In view of the societal and ecological consequences of energy production, energy policy requires broad public discussion and purposeful participation by citizens in the appropriate decisions. In the past, energy policy has been one-sidedly determined by economic considerations; only the protests of Burgerinitiativen have brought about a certain correction of this tendency. In the meantime, the interest in protecting nature and the environment is being more strongly taken into consideration in energy-policy discussions.

        In the near future, greater emphasis should be given to ways in which the views and interests of organizations concerned with protecting nature and the environment can become more important in energy-policy decision making. Groups of Burgerinitiativen and other organizations involved in environmental protection should thus be allowed to make their views heard in parliamentary hearings and to challenge the representatives of the responsible ministries and subordinate authorities to comment publicly and to answer important questions of detail.

As far as the construction of nuclear power plants is concerned, a responsible energy policy furthermore requires forward-looking planning of sites as well as a politically responsible policy of precaution for sites. The prevailing practice by which utility companies carry out the planning of sites leads to a problematical preference for energy economic and industry-economic considerations at the expense of ecological requirements and requirements of the proper allocation of space. Finally, the economically senseless result of this procedure has been that as much energy has been used as could be produced.

Site planning should be integrated into a procedure for ordering space, the political responsibility of which would be made apparent by procedures for discussion and explanation as well as by public hearings with appropriate journalistic and party-political evaluations of the controversies. Citizens' participation here, however, should not be realized by only the manufacture of publicity in the form of debates between the parties, discussion in the mass media, or spontaneous reactions by Burgerinitiativen. Beyond that, an organized participation by means of committees could make sense. While a site plan is being drawn up, these committees should participate according to §7 of the Landscape Law of North-Rhine Westphalia, which provides for committees to be formed "for the independent representation of the interests of nature and the landscape."

Attention certainly must be paid to make certain that these committees possess actual influence and do not atrophy into a new variation of interest-group pluralism. It is conceivable, for example, that the committee, to which representatives of the Burgerinitiative-federations and nature and environmental-protection groups should belong, should receive the right of a delaying veto.

Citizens' participation in environmental and energy-policy decisions on the one hand improves the objective basis upon which these decisions are to be made intelligently. On the other hand, it contributes to that from which democracy ultimately lives: the citizens' insight and trust in the legitimacy and responsibility of political decisions.

NOTES

(1)   Compare moreover Gaston Thorn: "Die Beeinflussung des
      politischen Entscheidungsprozesses entfallt dem Parlament
      in wesentlichen Bereichen und wird fortan von besser
      angepassten Interessengruppierungen . . . wahrgenom-
      men, die direkten Zugang zu der Regierung und den
      Verwaltungen haben und der Vermittlung durch das
      Parlament immer weniger bedurfen"; from his paper on
      the theme "Welche Zukunft hat die parlamentarische
      Demokratie westlicher Pragung?" in the Bergdorf
      discussion, here cited according to the Protocol, no. 51,
      Hamburg, 1975, p. 10.
(2)   The term originates from Gotz Briefs; see Ferdinand A.
      Hermens, Verfassungslehre, Frankfurt, 1964, p. 195.
(3)   Compare with Thomas Ellwein, Regieren und Verwalten,
      Opladen, 1976, p. 71. See also Gaston Thorn, op. cit.,
      p. 8: "Das Parlament wurde - zumindest in der Augen
      vieler - zu einer Kulisse degradiert, vor der - oder
      besser hinter der - die Schachzuge der Parteiapparate
      stattfinden."
(4)   For the problem of party financing in this connection,
      compare Uwe Schleth, Parteifinanzen, Meisenheim am
      Glahn 1973, p. 323; on the question of the social
      structure of the parties, see Karl-Heinz Nassmacher,
      "Parteien im kommunalpolitischen Zielbildungsprozess," in
      Osterreichische Zeitschrift fur Politikwissenschaft, vol. 1,
      no. 4, p. 51-59.

4 Participation in Energy Policy

Heino Galland

The energy policy in the Federal Republic of Germany is marked by a contradiction. On the one hand, numerous and extensive demands for participation in energy policy are registered, and the targets of such demands themselves require the legitimation of planning that participation could provide. On the other hand, completely insufficient possibilities for participation presently exist. This situation leads to the question of possibilities for change, for the innovation of social structures and institutions in this area.

The energy program of the Federal Republic and the partial programs appertaining to it have been subject to a process of rapid change since 1973. The processes of its formation and implementation have, for the most part, not yet received scientific analysis. Knowledge of previous programs, however, suggests that these processes are dominated by technocracy, i.e., by a coalition of industrial and scientific interests. Technocracy largely structures administrative decisions in advance, leaving little possibility of participation by the constitutional organs of decision. A gap thus arises between the constitutional organs and the population, a gap which widens when citizens complain of injury to their interests and demand direct participation in the processes of planning and decision.

Such demands flare up primarily in regard to the planning of energy-technical projects (project planning, regional planning) and subsequently sometimes regarding the planning of energy programs (program planning, national planning). They arise at the level of municipal institutions and involve decision makers up to the level of the Lander (states). A series of models of participation in other areas of politics, particularly city planning, the organization of the infrastructure, and location of industry, have been developed and in part institutionalized at this level. The possibilities for participation that this provides are regarded as completely insufficient.

At the level of program planning, possibilities for participation hardly extend beyond the familiar procedures of interest-group lobbying. Technocracy here shares the familiar problems of direct democracy in mass society. The scientific-industrial complex has largely monopolized information relevant to decision making and thus has structured essential decisions in advance. An investigation of the preconditions for participation must, therefore, first of all take account of the two levels of planning, project and program planning. At both levels, differing but mutually conditioning phases of planning take place. Planners and those affected by planning must keep sight of the system of planning as a whole.

The question of preconditions for participation can then be elucidated through examination of the structures and determining factors of the various phases of planning.

In particular, discussion must take the following directions:

1.   The structure of the energy-policy field must be analyzed in comparison to those fields of politics regarded as classical participatory domains. The central point in this analysis is the relation of state administration to private, semipublic, and public enterprises in the energy sector.
2.   There must follow an inquiry into the phases of planning at both planning levels.
3.   Upon this basis, determinants and factors which are essential to the introduction and operation of forms and models of participation must be investigated. This should make possible a systematic answer to the question of the applicability of participatory models to the energy field.
4.   Empirically investigated processes of participation, institutionalized models, and proposals and demands from the scientific and political communities must be analyzed and evaluated in light of the previously acquired insights.
5.   The more wide-reaching considerations that follow and extend beyond the narrow issue of participation should be discussed.

Points 1 and 4 require closer examination here than do the others. First, evidence will be presented that previously known forms of participation are not logically applicable to the problematic questions of energy planning. Second, from the demonstration of a connection between technocracy and bureaucracy, points of reference will be advanced for a strategy of action which, on the one hand, opens possibilities of direct action for the great majority of participants and concerned parties and, on the other, promises to affect the actual processes of planning.

POLITICAL STRUCTURES

In the political system of the Federal Republic of Germany, the traditional field of participatory politics is that of municipal policy. The reasons for this are the following:

1. Municipal autonomy as an essential precondition of participation is the result of long-range, historical decision-making processes. Here one must note, however, that the factual, and frequently in consequence, formal decision-making jurisdiction of the municipalities can no longer be covered by the concept of municipal autonomy. This is due to political centralization of the state, which is in turn a consequence of economic developments.

2. Municipal policy is the political field in which politics can be actually experienced to the greatest extent. This is true of political decision makers, institutions, and administrative facilities as well as of the inputs and outputs of the municipal political system.

3. The perception by citizens that interests are positively or negatively affected by decisions and planning is relatively widespread.

4. This perception is decisively increased through the participation of economic interests, especially in relation to infrastructure and location of new industry.

5. The municipality, as the smallest entity of the political system, presents the lowest degree of complexity for the formation of public opinion. Thus, for example, conditional interconnections are most easily detected, and thus frustration as a consequence of insufficient clarity of political processes is lowest.

6. Professional competence of municipal employees is highest due to career experience and other knowledge of planning processes.

With these structural characteristics, the municipality is the political entity most genuinely favorable to participation. Does this stand in contrast to the relationships of politics and economics in the municipal sector? Here one must distinguish between economic groups and areas of decision.

Industry's interest in municipal politics concentrates essentially on questions of the location of new industry, infrastructure policies, and economic promotion (the construction industry and related fields are an exception). Otherwise, the representation of industrial interests begins essentially at the federal level.

Particularly in the field of infrastructure policy, demands upon the municipality are differing and in part contradictory because of varying conditions for the reproduction of capital and labor. This creates relatively greater scope for action by the organs of decision. Even when the community economic structure sets essential conditions for municipal policy and when economic groups help determine certain essential aspects of that policy, considerable leeway still remains for a labor-oriented municipal policy.

On the other hand, enterprises in the tertiary sector (trade, commerce, services) are often closely interwoven with municipal policy and considerably influence, inter alia, policies toward infrastructure and the location of industry. Thus, the community's leeway in these matters is generally limited. Jobs, taxes, and purchasing power are usually the decisive factors.

If the relationship of politics to the economy (particularly industry) in the local community can generally be termed rather loose, the possibilities for institutionalized participation appear, on this basis, likely to be realized. This does not mean that familiar forms of participation in the municipality are effective, since impediments to effective participation lie not only in certain relations between politics and economics, but also in the political system itself. Here more structural, systemically conditioned impediments must be distinguished from those which are accidental or which stem from the peculiarities of a particular issue.

THE STRUCTURE OF THE ENERGY-POLICY FIELD

One must first note that the social sciences, aside from a portion of economic science, have only concerned themselves with energy policy since around 1974. Systematic works are appearing gradually, and only a very few works seem reliable and of lasting value. The relation between political science and energy policy is still characterized by a considerable deficit of empirical knowledge, which is manifested in the mediocre quality of theorization in this area.

In the domain of energy-project planning, energy policy and municipal policy share certain points of contact. The traditional municipal jurisdiction over the site of energy-technology projects is considerably reduced, however, by preliminary steps in planning and decision making taken by corporations, Lander, and the federal government. The complexity of the phases of planning reflects complexity of the technology involved. The leeway for decision making by municipalities in the location of energy-technical projects is, therefore, smaller than in other infrastructural planning.

The microeconomic considerations for location of such projects are primarily these: location vis-a-vis the high-voltage electrical network; location vis-a-vis major concentrations of consumers; geology of the site; factors involved in the cooling process; and prospects for authorization, or expected length of the process of obtaining authorization.

The major consideration for federal and Lander authorization should be these: safety of the facility for employees, residents, and surroundings; questions of space and of conservation; and energy needs and possibilities of meeting them. In the judgment of those affected by planning, governmental authorizations frequently ignore these criteria.

Last-minute decisions result to a great extent in the selection of sites which cannot easily be changed through the formation of public opinion on a local level. If the community's scope for action concerning location of new industry is already rather small, it shrinks even further in the case of energy-technical facilities. The leeway for political participation is too small.

In the case of atomic power stations, a new, central factor is the problem of perceiving and evaluating risks. Decisions involving such great uncertainty demand the opportunity for participation. The planning process permits little scope for participation, however. In this contradictory situation, open conflict is the frequent consequence. (This line of argument must be further developed: the question must be considered whether decisions on site location can practically be made in earlier phases of planning.)

Contradictory hypotheses have been developed concerning the relationship between politics and economics in the energy sector:

1. State energy policy is dependent on micro-economic and sectoral planning;(1)
2. The energy sector is an example of extensive state influence in guiding investment decisions;(2) and
3. State activity in the energy field is largely ineffective and frequently arbitrary.

It is generally agreed that, in practice, a high degree of interconnection exists between politics and economics in energy planning. It has thus become questionable whether a conceptual and factual dichotomy between these two sectors still exists.

The theoretical and empirical clarification of the relationship between politics and economics in the energy field is an essential prerequisite for analysis. It provides the answer to the question of whether or not there is a place for public participation in energy planning. Only when this is clarified does a response to the question of the possibilities for participation make sense.

At the level of project planning one must trace the course of planning and empirically determine the relationship between politics and economics by systematizing disparate experiences and information.

The level of state program planning appears empirically clearer. Analyses are available of the formation and significance of older partial programs (e.g., atomic programs, coal adaptation plans). If one can assume the economic necessity of state program planning, at the same time one can confirm only very conditionally the relevance of energy policy programs to economic processes in the energy field.

The early phases of energy programs show a high dependence of state planning upon the delivery of economic data on energy. The phases of implementation, on the other hand, exhibit a high degree of arbitrary state activity.

Political science's theoretical questions concerning program planning cannot at present be answered precisely. Possibilities for answers to these questions would seem to lie within the range of hypotheses 1 and 3. Newer partial programs of the federal and Lander governments show a tendency to use, albeit with some hestitation, the resource of participation and provide evidence to support hypothesis 2. The lack of planning of state responsibilities and insufficient coordination of program planning have negative consequences for program planning itself and indicate, moreover, the absence of participation.

A preliminary summary would list a series of differences in the structures of the energy policy and municipal policy fields:

o   The nature and extent of entanglement between politics and economics are qualitatively different. The degree of autonomy of state action in the energy sector is smaller;

o   The complexity of the planning processes is qualitatively different;

o   Further differences and peculiarities exist, such as the varying degree to which planning can be determined, dif-ferences among decision-making situations under varying degrees of uncertainty, and the relationship among interest, motivation, and planning.

By no means all characteristics of the energy-policy field lead to the conclusion that forms of institutionalized participation have no prospects or are impossible. A series of peculiarities must be noted, however, which make participation in this field quite difficult to achieve. An extraordinary degree of social innovation is required to overcome the existing obstacles. This condition raises the question of empirically verifiable forms of participation.

EMPIRICALLY VERIFIABLE PARTICIPATORY BEHAVIOR

A knowledge of empirically verifiable forms of participation should make it possible to answer the question of what innovative powers can be mobilized and of what problems exist in the political utilization of such powers.

The information necessary for this analysis can be gained in four ways:

1. through state and private regulatory, informational, and security services;
2. through the mass media;
3. through empirical social and political research;
4. through statements of the actors involved.

The third and fourth methods appear the most legitimate means of obtaining valid information.

In empirical social and political research, one must distinguish between quantitative and qualitative methods. Standardized and structuralized polls are the primary quantitative methods in the survey field. These polling methods have often been utilized in the Federal Republic of Germany during the last several years.(3) The quality of results is frequently suspect, since this method may be ill-suited to questions in the energy field. The energy consciousness of the population is marked by

- a low degree of structure (uncertainty),
- a great degree of impulsive development (instability),
- a great dependence on knowledge of other political fields, and thus
- a high degree of difficulty quantifying information.

The complex traits of public consciousness of energy reflect the actual conditions of the energy sector; it is particularly complex because of the difficulty of comprehending highly complex technological issues.

This consciousness is essentially not measurable by the standard instruments of social research since questions on energy, unlike those on election or market surveys, can be worded in any conceivable number of ways. The great majority of efforts to determine public attitudes on energy have failed to formulate adequate questions. Completely contradictory results have been obtained because of the wording of the questions. Thus, statements of the type "X percent of the population favors primary energy source A" are generally useless. The nature of the questions is conditioned by factors that arise from the forms of organization of empirical social research, such as

- interests which influence results, particularly the interests of economic and political contractors;
- time and cost limitations on investigations;
- availability of research clarifies the problem which can lead to a more intense analysis of the question.

To simplify somewhat, quantitative assertions about the energy consciousness of the population are of little practical value. At best, the results of quantitative analysis can lead to very rough assessment of general trends, e.g., that the number of those favoring nuclear power plants has declined between 1974 and 1978.

Material on attitudes toward related areas (environment, state, economy, participation, education, etc.) provides a key to knowledge of the factors conditioning energy consciousness and its dynamism. On this basis, one can identify trends concerning the relationship between social class and other data provided by social statistics and trends concerning the attitudes toward questions relating to energy. The nature of these relationships is presented in detail in the reports "Burgerinitiativen im Bereich von Kernkraftwerken ("Citizens' Initiatives in the Field of Atomic Power Plants") and "Einstellung und Verhalten der Bervolkerung gegenuber verschiedenen Energiegewinnungsarten" ("Attitude and Behavior of the Population toward Various Means of Obtaining Energy"), and it will not be summarized here. Similarly conducted investigations concerning the relationships among sets of attitudes come to comparable conclusions (e.g., EMNIC, 1976).

Qualitative methods such as participatory observations, experts' discussions, and research activity generate different but no less serious problems: their results cannot be generalized; the process of data collection is less verifiable; and restrictions of time and cost often bear even more heavily upon the quality of the results than with other methods. This set of methods is strongest, however, at the level of project planning because of its recording of extensive complexes of attitudes and behavior.(4)

Empirical results concerning participatory behavior in the energy sector are of limited use without knowledge of energy consciousness and related matters. The accuracy of such results is limited by potential short-term changes, which greatly hinders the attempt to develop institutionalized methods of participation. What is clear, however, is that participatory behavior itself renders institutionalization difficult.(5) Forms of participation in the energy sector are largely marked by open conflict between planners and those affected by planning. This conflict results in part from the absence of possibilities for participation; it is caused also by the extreme length of the preliminary periods for planning. The effect of both factors together is that those affected must endure technocratic planning without the opportunity for democratic legitimation. Mistrust, hostility, suspicion, and severe disturbances of communication characterize the situation, and open conflicts are the most unfavorable situations imaginable for institutionalized participation. Nonetheless, openly conducted conflicts can represent preliminary stages for the establishment of new adjustment mechanisms.

Furthermore, the social and political structures of the concerned groups are extraordinarily heterogeneous. These groups achieve homogeneity almost exclusively as "single-issue movements" (e.g., when such a group forms to object to a single, specific project, such as the construction of a particular nuclear plant). At the same time, the dynamism of the conflict has led to an explosive broadening of the contents and objectives of the ecology movement, which has split into several different divisions. One must differentiate, for example, among a conservative-agrarian-conservationist group, a strong group of disappointed members and supporters of the government parties (SPD and FDP) and of the unions, a stronger socialist-ecological group, a spontaneous, action-oriented group, and a group which directly practices alternative life-styles. Of course, the boundaries between these groupings are fluid. Corrsponding to the heterogeneity of the groups and their objectives is their plethora of political tactics and differing conceptions of solutions to conflicts. But only those procedures that develop from the practical controversy and are based on as broad a consensus as possible have a chance of being institutionalized.

The course of conflicts over energy policy is also characterized by a lengthy, continuing and, in part, intentionally impeded search for the correct target for demands. In other words, concerned persons who attempt to participate in the field of energy policy and experience the entanglement of politics and economics, which, as joint foci of the planning process, are the principal targets of demands for greater participation.(6) In the course of conflict, however, the attempt is often made to shove the responsibility for

planning onto someone else. (For example, the Ministry of
Research and Technology has said, "We build no atomic power
plants.") This dodging of responsibility results in frustration
for those concerned and can discourage their further
cooperation.

The participation of external groups in the investment
decisions of private enterprises is - at least as far as certain
industrial and political dogmatists are concerned - contrary to
the rules of the system. The participatory rights of internal
groups, especially of dependent employees, are extremely
narrow in this respect and are practically limited to obtaining
information. The possibilities for state involvement generally
extend no further than to decisions affecting the overall legal,
financial, and economic milieu. For there to be effective forms
of participation in corporate planning, there must be developed
new models of microeconomic decision making, a field which has
been explored except for some preliminary discussions in the
SPD in connection with what was at the time called its
long-term program.

The level of state program planning also displays no
inclination toward the institutionalization of participation.
Already-institutionalized rights relate mostly to consultation,
hearings, and advance information privileges for certain
affected highly institutionalized interest groups. Participation
here, too, is considered contrary to the system.

The participatory behavior of planners and concerned
parties does not at present give cause for a prognosis for
institutionalization of greater participatory rights in the near
future. At the same time, the question remains of whether
new adjustment mechanisms might not develop, almost as a
natural growth, out of the present situations of conflict.

For the social sciences, a fundamental restriction of
developing models of participation remains because of the
problems of empirical methods of measuring participatory
behavior.

THE INSTITUTIONALIZATION OF PARTICIPATION

There have been a few attempts to overcome the difficulties
involved in participation in energy policy:

1. at the level of project planning, there has been
    discussion of the right of grievance of interest
    groups and, in this connection, discussion of
    the question of counterevaluations;
2. at the level of program planning, there have
    been the "citizens' dialogue on atomic energy"
    and the proposals of the Battelle Research
    group.

Neither of these attempts is suited to maintaining the precarious balance between the contrary interests of those involved in the planning process. The interest group's so-called right of grievance is a basic demand of those affected by planning. That it needs to be discussed reflects the sort of governmental attitudes that result, for example, in property rights being accorded more consideration than the demands of organizations which represent entire population groups.(7)

Among groups of concerned persons, controversy continues regarding the group grievance. The demand is supported by sections of the government parties and by numerous scientists. Such a proposal is set forth, inter alia, in the report Burgerinitiativen im Bereich von Kernkraft-werken."(8) Numerous conceptions have been developed of what the concrete form of the group grievance should be. As usual, the details present the greatest difficulties.(9) Even weakened variants have hitherto been criticized by the government parties as offering too many possibilities for a blockade of all planning. One should also note that even without a group's right of grievance, a number of judicial proceedings have been delayed a long while, which resulted in increased costs and other factors leading to a termination of planning.

In these proceedings, plaintiffs for the group must contend with numerous disadvantages. The significance of the group's grievance does not lie primarily in its effect upon the outcome of trials, which are more strongly influenced by other factors, and its significance lies little or not at all in its effects on the results of planning. Rather, its importance lies primarily in its reduction of the groups' disadvantages against private individuals in judicial proceedings. The groups' right of grievance cannot, however, create equal "firing power" on both sides. Large, highly specialized administrative bodies in government, business, and the scientific community prevail almost without exception over far greater, though often in some respects more selective, professional expertise.

The demand for counterevaluations stems from the enormous gap in access to information. A corresponding proposal is contained in the report " Burgerinitiativen im Bereich von Kernkraftwerken." It calls for the establishment by the authorizing authorities of a .5 million DM fund (.03 percent of the construction costs of 1.5 billion DM), to be jointly administered by the authorities and by plaintiffs. A problem here is how plaintiffs are to be recognized or registered by the authorizing authorities. The question of counterevaluations includes three principal problems:

o   expert evaluators must be found;
o   they must have adequate work conditions; and
o   they must be paid.

The economic power of the opposing side gives it an advantage in dealing with all three of these problems.

Even both proposals taken together do not eliminate the completely asymmetrical relations of power. That nothing to ameliorate the imbalance has as yet been undertaken reflects the extraordinarily strong concentration and consolidation of power on the side of industry and government. Attempts at a solution are thus not to be sought exclusively, or primarily, at the level of project planning.

It is problematic in a discussion of the problems of participation to allude to the "Burgerdialog Kernenergie" (citizens' dialogue on atomic energy) of the Ministry of Research and Technology. The participatory value of this "citizens' dialogue" is generally considered to be quite low. On the other hand, the dialogue is the first attempt at organized, open communication on the level of program planning. The citizens' dialogue contains the following elements:

● engaging in traditional public relations work of the Ministry, such as publications, advertisements, brochures;
● participating in public events (forum discussions, weekend seminars);
● preparing special brochures, documentations, circular letters;
● arranging and financing external events (conferences, etc.);
● conveying information, addresses, names of experts, etc.;
● financing organizations; and
● publishing state-of-the-art reports.

The best known activities are those involving the least amount of participation. This fact has contributed to the poor public image of the citizens' dialogue. The most useful activities are little known, but they represent an important aid to the political involvement of concerned parties.

The citizens' dialogue is structurally removed from planning at the project and the program levels. This has been both the intention of its initiators and a central point of criticism of participants. At the same time, concerned individuals and groups have new and better possibilities for articulation through the help of the citizens' dialogue. Changes in the budget of the Research Ministry (energy research program) illustrate the influence, albeit limited, of the energy discussion upon the Ministry's planning.

The discussion of the possibility of participation in energy policy has uncovered a large number of difficulties. The structures of the respective political fields are very different. The empirically verifiable forms of participation have yet to be institutionalized. Proposals and attempts to broaden participation by citizens either lack participatory substance or have been stalled at the level of political decision making.

On this basis, a provisional prognosis must state that open conflict over energy policy will continue and that a transition to new adjustment mechanisms is not yet in sight. Nonetheless, in view of the central difficulty - on the one hand, there is a great need for participation, and, on the other hand, there are minimal possibilities for it - the task of participation research remains to seek ways of changing the existing processes of planning.

NOTES

(1) Karsten Pruss, Kerforschungspolitik in der Bundes-republik Deutschland (Frankfurt, 1974), pp. 38-44.

(2) Bundesministerium fur Forschung und Technologie, Einstellungen und Verhalten der Bevolkerung gegenuber verschiedenen Energiegewinnungsarten, volume II: Materialen. June 1977, pp. 2-8 (cited as "Einstellungen und Verhalten").

(3) Most of these investigations have not been published because of the forms of organization of empirical social research. Thus they cannot be discussed individually at this point.

(4) E.g., Theodor Ebert, Wolfgang Sternstein, Roland Vogt, Okologiebewegung und Ziviler Widerstand. Wyhler Er-fahrungen. Aktionsforscher berichten.

(5) As a case study see: Bundesministerium fur Forschung and Technologie (publisher): Burgerinitiativen im Bereich von Kernkraftwerken (Munich, 1975).

(6) Einstellungen und Verhalten, volume 2, pp. 2-3.

(7) Peter Cornelius Meyer-Tasch, "Burgerinitiativen und verwaltungsgerichtlicher Rechtsschutz - Ein Beitrag zur Rechtsproblematik der Burgerinitiativen," in Burger-beteiligung und Burgerinitiativen ed. Hans Matthofer (Villingen, 1977), p. 213-221.

(8) Burgerinitiativen, pp. 313-316 (counterevaluations, p. 314 ff.).

(9) Eckart Rehbinder, "Moglichkeit, Notwendigkeit und Zweckmassigkeit einer Klagebefugnis fur private Um-weltorganisationwn." Gutachten fur den Bundesminister des Innern. (Frankfurt, 1974): Unveroffentlichte Manuskripte.

5 Citizens' Participation at Government Expense

Joan B. Aron

Within the past few years, scholarly journals and the media have paid marked attention to alternative measures for promoting participation in regulatory decision making as a step toward regulatory reform.(1) Notwithstanding the limited success of these measures in bringing previously un-represented points of view into the formulation of regulatory decisions, a common theme emerges: How can interested citizen groups gain sufficient technical expertise and professional knowledge to compete successfully with industry representatives?

The question becomes more critical when one considers that the public hearing - "the administrative proceeding at which the record is compiled,...policy is refined and conflicting interests are ultimately resolved"(2) - is the primary forum for the input of citizens to and feedback from the regulatory process. Yet Schuck points out that "it is at this point that public interest groups are at their most conspicuous disadvantage."(3) Even if groups of citizens have sufficient access to participate in an agency's decision-making process, they still need technical and legal information, time, and resources to participate effectively. Despite agreement by many observers that a possible solution would be to compensate citizens' groups for their use of legal and technical consultants, there has been little optimism on this score. Paglin and Shor found that federal regulatory bodies had made "conspicuously inconsistent responses" in providing direct financial assistance to citizens' groups that intervened in agency proceedings and that the agencies which dealt with complex technical issues were less apt to be receptive than agencies having consumer-protection re-sponsibilities.(4) Moreover, Paglin and Shor, foreseeing protracted debate and indefinite delays before the adoption of financial aid and programs, were not optimistic about the possibility of gaining a more positive reception for requests for such assistance.

Nevertheless, signs of change are visible in all sectors of the government. With the advent of the Carter administration, a new group of administrators and regulatory commissioners took office who have different perspectives from those who were displaced. Their views have been reflected and, in some cases, institutionalized in new agency procedures and programs for financing consumer groups. Although Congress once again rejected the proposal for the creation of a consumer-protection agency, an instrument strongly favored by the new administration for the presentation of consumer interests in regulatory proceedings, the demise of the consumer agency for the near future at least may have provided the impetus for resorting to more radical measures for protecting consumer interests.(5) The administration has included a section on limited funding for the participation of eligible groups in the regulatory process in proposed legislation S.755, the Regulation Reform Act of 1979 (introduced March 26, 1979).

If the provision of direct financing to citizens' groups, commonly called intervenor funding, is gaining general acceptance within the executive establishment, it warrants closer scrutiny than it has received in the past. Is direct financing a reasonable way to facilitate participation in the regulatory process? Does it serve the needs of the interested public and regulatory agencies? What are the perceived benefits and costs of the new procedures? Who should receive the funds? What can we learn from federal experience? Are the rules of the regulatory process such that intervention will be accepted? Finally, does the new procedure provide a genuine opportunity to influence agency policy or is it merely a token encouragement of the outsider's point of view?

SIGNS OF CHANGE IN THE PUBLIC SECTOR

In the past year, federal agencies have undertaken a large number of unilateral initiatives to fund intervenors in agency proceedings. At least ten agencies have issued rule-making proposals calling for the reimbursement of participants' expenses. Among these agencies are the Food and Drug Administration (FDA), the Environmental Protection Agency (EPA), the National Highway Traffic Safety Administration (NHTSA), the Consumer Product Safety Commission (CPSC), the Federal Trade Commission (FTC), the National Oceanic and Atmospheric Administration (NOAA), the Department of Commerce, the Civil Aeronautics Board (CAB), and the Federal Communications Commission (FCC). In addition, both the

Department of Interior and the Department of Agriculture have
published notices that they are considering the reimbursement
of intervenor expenses.   Although the FTC, EPA, and NHTSA
are the only agencies that thus far have some experience in
implementing the new procedures, it is fair to assume that
more will follow their lead.

Interestingly, despite the gloomy prognostications about
the relative unwillingness of hardware-oriented agencies, those
dealing with complex technological issues, to implement
intervenor funding, the evidence seems to point in the other
direction.   The three major federal agencies dealing with
energy regulation have displayed a recent awareness of the
need to provide financial support to consumer groups.   The
Department of Energy has made grants to consumer groups in
three proceedings, and it has announced its intention of
drafting regulations to provide support for such groups to
participate in rule-making and policy-development activities.(6)
The Federal Energy Regulatory Commission (FERC), successor
to the Federal Power Commission, has also expressed a desire
to provide compensation for expenses of intervenors in its
proceedings, and it has received statutory authority to do
so.(7)   The Nuclear Regulatory Commission (NRC), which had
terminated consideration of rules to provide assistance to
participants in Commission proceedings in 1976, included a
section on intervenor funding in draft legislation on nuclear
licensing reform provided to the administration in September
1978.   The NRC also supported the administration's proposal
for funding intervenors that was contained in the licensing
bills (H.R.11704 and S.2775) which were introduced (but not
passed) in the 95th Congress.

There is some legal uncertainty about the agencies'
authority to spend federal funds for intervenor reimbursement.
Recent rulings by the Comptroller General and the courts have
furnished conflicting guidance to agencies concerning the
expenditure of agency funds for this purpose in the absence
of specific Congressional authorization.   In a few cases,
Congressional permission has been given.   The Magnuson-Moss
Warranty Act (P.L. 93-637, 1975) authorizes the FTC to
provide compensation for reasonable attorneys' fees, expert
witnesses' fees, and other costs to individuals and citizens'
groups for participating in rule-making proceedings.   The
Toxic Substances Control Act (P.L. 94-469, 1976) extends
similar authorization to EPA for use in certain rule-making
proceedings.   The Utility Regulatory Policies Act of 1978 (P.L.
95-617) permits financial assistance to persons intervening in
FERC's proceedings.

In other instances, concerned federal agencies have
sought legal advice from the Comptroller General concerning
their authority to provide financial assistance for participation.   The rulings have been consistently favorable.   The

Comptroller General advised the FTC in 1972 that the
Commission had inherent authority to use appropriated funds
to reimburse indigent parties and intervenors for attorneys'
fees and other costs incurred in regulatory proceedings.(8)
Similarly, he advised the NRC in 1976 that it had the statutory
authority to reimburse financially needy intervenors when the
Commission believed such participation was "essential" to
represent opposing points of view (B-92288, February 19,
1976). Subsequently, the Comptroller General extended his
finding on NRC to eight other regulatory agencies (FCC, FPC,
ICC, CPSC, SEC, FDA, EPA, and NHTSA) on the condition
that no specific statutory prohibition was present (B-180224,
May 10, 1976).

The Comptroller General has also moved to liberalize the
criteria for intervenor funding set forth in the advice to the
NRC. In response to the FDA, the Comptroller General ruled
that the expenses of needy participants in all types of agency
proceedings might be reimbursed when their participation could
"reasonably be expected to contribute substantially to a full
and fair determination" of pending issues. He also stated that
the participation need not be "essential" in the sense that the
issues could be decided without it (B-139703, December 3,
1976).

Notwithstanding the Comptroller General's opinions, the
courts have displayed an ambivalent view toward financial
assistance for participation. In a series of disputes between
the Greene County Planning Board and the Federal Power
Commission in which the FPC consistently took the position
that it lacked power to pay intervenors' costs in the absence
of explicit statutory authority, the courts have in turn
sustained and then overruled the agency's point of view. In
the most recent case, argued in 1978, a majority of the U.S.
Court of Appeals overruled a previous court order calling for
reimbursement of needy intervenors by the FPC, holding that
the Commission's authority to disburse funds must come from
Congress. The decision also stated that it was the court's
responsibility, rather than that of the Comptroller General, to
determine the legislative intent of Congress.(9)

Events subsequent to the Greene County decisions appear
to confirm the tendency of federal regulatory agencies, noted
earlier, to shift opinion on intervenor funding. For example,
the FERC has disavowed the FPC's traditional view that it
lacks statutory authority to fund expenses of needy parties in
agency proceedings and has sought reconsideration of the
Greene County decision by the Supreme Court.(10) Another
sequel to the Greene County cases came in the form of an
advisory opinion from the U.S. Attorney General to DOT
and CAB stating that the Greene County decision related
only to the Federal Power Act and that "no department or
agency . . . other than possibly FERC is bound by that

holding."(11)   A recent federal district court opinion permitted
the U.S. Department of Agriculture to fund, by contract,
participation by a consumer group in a study of the impact of
proposed labeling regulations.   Like the Attorney General, the
court held that the Greene County decision was based largely
on the FPC's aversion to funding intervenors and its singular
construction of its statutory authority.(12)

CONGRESSIONAL ACTIVITIES

Congress took no action during the 94th and 95th sessions on
two key bills, S.2715 and S.270, both of which provide for
"Public Participation in Federal Agency Proceedings."
Nevertheless, there is reason to believe that the concept of
intervenor funding is gaining momentum in Congress.   Both
these bills, sponsored by Senator Kennedy, would have
authorized federal regulatory bodies to award the fees and
costs of experts and other costs of participation to eligible
persons in rule making, rate making, licensing, and other
types of proceedings.   Although the Senate Judiciary
Committee has heretofore failed to act on the bills, this year
Senator Kennedy is chairman of the Committee, the composition
of which has changed, and there is reason to believe the
concept of intervenor assistance is likely to receive a more
positive reception.
        There has been further evidence of Congressional support
for intervenor funding.   In 1976, the House Subcommittee on
Oversight and investigations of the Committee on Interstate
and Foreign Commerce explored the practices of the regulatory
commissions and executive agencies under its jurisdiction and
recommended direct agency funding of citizens' groups as a
"means of improving public participation in regulatory
decision-making processes."(13)   The Senate Committee on
Governmental Affairs conducted a comprehensive six-volume
study of federal regulation and expressed this notion more
strongly.   The Committee found that "the single greatest
obstacle to active public participation in regulatory proceedings
is the lack of financial resources by potential participants to
meet the great costs of formal participation"; it recommended
Congressional enactment of "legislation authorizing compensation to eligible persons."(14)   To this end, the Committee introduced legislation, S.262, the Reform of Federal
Regulation Act of 1979 (January 31, 1979), which provides for
financial assistance to qualified intervenors in agency
proceedings.
        The Senate Committee also recommended that "until
such time as general legislation for compensation of public

participation costs is enacted, regulatory agencies should implement their own programs . . . as appropriate."(15)

PERCEIVED BENEFITS OF INTERVENOR FUNDING

The recent trend in support of intervenor funding reflects an apparent presumption by the affected governmental bodies that they will derive benefits from such an additional expenditure of public funds. What in fact do the federal agencies expect to gain by the adoption of this practice?

The perceived benefits of intervenor funding have received more attention than the possible disadvantages. The former can be summarized and categorized as follows.

The need to reduce the imbalance in participation by industry and citizens' groups at regulatory proceedings is an important factor underlying support for intervenor funding. The Senate Committee on Governmental Affairs found that public participation was extremely limited, stating that

> At agency after agency, participation by the regulated industry predominates - often over-whelmingly. . . . In more than half of the formal proceedings, there appears to be no . . . (organized public interest) participation whatsoever and virtually none at informal agency proceedings. In those proceedings where participation by public groups does take place, typically it is a small fraction of the participation by the regulated industry. One-tenth is not uncommon; sometimes it is even less than that.(16)

Moreover, the Committee found a tremendous disparity in expenditures for participation by industry and public-interest groups, noting that "the regulated industry consistently out-spends public participants by a wide margin."(17) In nuclear licensing proceedings, for example, where the costs of specialized counsel and expert witnesses are unusually large, the Committee estimated that industry expenditures typically ranged from $500,000-1,000,000, or ten to twenty times more than a public-interest group could afford to spend in contesting a license.(18)

Another argument in support of intervenor funding relies on the notion that citizen-participants with competing viewpoints would provide decision makers with a broader range of alternative considerations to reach a balanced judgment. Hence, administrators and staff would be more sensitive to the concerns of an enlarged number of constituencies in discharging their public responsibilities. It is believed that broader participation would curb the typical industry orientation of regulatory bodies in at least four ways: "it would present decision makers with new ideas and information, reduce their dependence on data supplied by the regulated industry, compel them to seek an accommodation with new groups, and aid in the development of a more comprehensive record."(19)

Intervenor funding is also supported by the widespread belief that involvement by citizens in litigation has had a significant and salutary effect on making regulatory decisions. Judge Harold Leventhal of the U.S. Court of Appeals, District of Columbia, points out:

> Administrative law and regulation has been profoundly influenced by the participation, in agencies and in court, of the public interest representation. They have identified issues and caused agencies and courts to look squarely at problems that would otherwise have been swept aside and passed unnoticed. They have made complaints, adduced and martialed evidence, offered different insights and viewpoints, and presented scientific, historical and legal research.(20)

Documentation for these assertions is extensive and covers many areas of regulatory activity. To cite just one example, drawn from the field of nuclear power, an Atomic Safety Licensing and Appeals Board has commented:

> The development of plant security requirements were influenced considerably by the probing questions of CCPE's (Citizens Concerned with the Protection of the Environment) counsel. . . . This constructive participation on an important issue has, in our judgment, contributed to the improvement of the regulatory process, both as an aid to the adjudication of the security issues and in the development of the overall regulatory requirements in an evolving area.(21)

Although intervention by public-interest groups is commonly believed to be a major cause of delay in regulatory proceedings, many first-hand observers disagree. The participation of diverse parties may tend to leave litigants more satisfied with the results of administrative decisions and, therefore, obviate further appeal to the courts. From this point of view, the implementation of intervenor funding might provide less of a burden on the courts' appellate procedures over the long run than at first seems likely. Confirming this idea, the Senate Committee on Governmental Affairs notes that:

"Ultimately, . . . the overall time elapsed may in fact be lessened, since if all relevant issues are resolved in the initial proceeding, the likelihood of a subsequent court reversal to consider relevant issues is substantially reduced, and along with it the risk that the agency will simply have to go through its paces all over again."(22)

Finally, it is alleged that enlarged citizen participation, facilitated by intervenor funding, would contribute to public information and public education about the issues raised in regulatory proceedings. Hence, public confidence in regulatory decisions would be enhanced. This argument holds that proceedings which deal with complex, technical, and controversial issues, which are not easily comprehended by the general public, would meet with greater acceptance from broader public exposure.(23) It seems clear that decisions arrived at in an open participatory forum - with access allowed to all interested parties - would elicit a higher degree of public confidence than those which are made by a small, select group behind closed doors.

PERCEIVED DISADVANTAGES OF INTERVENOR FUNDING

The alleged disadvantages of intervenor funding are in large measure the reverse of those characteristics that are cited as benefits. Like the supposed benefits, they are speculative in nature and concern the following issues.

Opponents of intervenor funding claim that the practice would encourage irresponsible participation at regulatory proceedings, create deadlocks in the decision-making process, and add to the workload of regulatory agencies and appeal tribunals. In this way, regulatory proceedings which are already long and unwieldy might become even more prolonged.

For example, Joseph Swidler, former chairman of the Federal Power Commission and the New York Public Service Commission, has testified that

> The crucial problems in public administration today are the growing backlogs, the inability to accord prompt justice, and in some areas an inability to act which borders upon paralysis of the regulatory structure. Far from a lack of private intervenors to represent the public interest in their own fashion, the last decade has witnessed an enormous proliferation of such intervenors, with which the regulatory agencies have not yet learned to cope. It is this factor as much as any other which has slowed down the agencies in the dispatch of their work. . . . The situation would be worse,

much worse (if intervenor funding were to be adopted).(24)

Another counterargument is based on the belief that top administrators and staff of public agencies are charged with responsibility for representing the public interest and already possess the requisite expertise and resources to do so adequately. From this point of view, intervenor funding would merely enable outside groups that are not accountable to a representative constituency to perform (less well) the same work as the regulatory staff.(25) This argument is buttressed by the notion that regulatory proceedings already contain ample opportunities for public intervention. Therefore, further expenditures of public funds to enhance participation by outside groups would be wasteful.

Opponents believe also that the adoption of intervenor funding on a governmentwide basis should be preceded by a thoroughgoing appraisal of the programs in existence. Since some programs are already under way, they believe it would be sensible to evaluate the experience at hand and to take corrective action if appropriate.(26)

Another counterclaim is that participating groups would be coopted by the regulatory agencies over the long run. According to this view, agencies with funding capabilities would tend to show favoritism toward persons or groups whom they know, who have testified effectively before the agency in the past, and who can be counted on to make arguments that the agency wishes to hear. The independence of the participating groups would therefore be undermined, the quality of the testimony would suffer, and the purpose of the intervention would be frustrated.(27)

FEDERAL EXPERIENCE WITH INTERVENOR FUNDING

Given the claims and counterclaims for intervenor funding, what can we learn from an examination of agency practice? We have noted that EPA, FTC, and NHTSA are the primary examples of agencies with statutory authority to finance intervenors in their proceedings. Of these, EPA has financed intervenor groups at only two hearings, and FTC has yet to evaluate its experience in a systematic way. Data relating to the FTC operation come from testimony presented at the Senate hearings on S.270, Public Participation in Federal Agency Proceedings Act, by the former chairman, Calvin J. Collier. At that time (February 1977), Mr. Collier pointed out that funding intervenors over a two-year period had yielded "substantial benefits" to FTC rule-making proceedings, enabling participants to develop and present factual evidence and research results at hearings on funeral costs, prescription drug advertising, hearing aids, and food advertising.(28)

As of February 1979, the FTC has spent nearly two million dollars in its funding program and has reimbursed nearly fifty persons or groups for their participation. It continues to believe that the program has been a "major success in improving the rulemaking process."(29)

More concrete evidence gained from federal experience comes from an evaluation of a one-year financial assistance demonstration program made by the National Highway Safety Administration (NHTSA) in 1977. The report was uniformly favorable, stating that the program had, among other things

- provided decision makers with broader understanding of the affected interests;
- enabled funding participants to make a meaningful contribution to rule-making procedures;
- ensured participation by informed and interested citizens;
- diminished the likelihood that organizations with high economic interests in the outcome would unduly influence the flow of information;
- diminished the possibility of judicial and legislative attack;
- produced relevant evidence and arguments and strengthened the administrative record; and
- not caused any substantial delays.

In conclusion, the evaluation found that compensating participants was feasible and "a valuable adjunct to existing rule-making procedures."(30) The report recommended extension of the program and application of intervenor funding on a departmentwide basis. Effective January 13, 1978, NHTSA's demonstration program was extended until further notice.

The lessons derived from federal experience can also provide a basis for identifying some of the ways to make intervenor funding a more effective tool in public participation.

Ample notice is useful. NHTSA suggested that "the need for adequate time for public announcement submission of applications, agency evaluation, participant preparation and presentation cannot be overstressed."(31) It warned that sufficient time was needed for these preliminary activities; otherwise, less well-established groups would be unlikely to hear of the availability of funding and compensated participants would have neither the time to formulate their arguments nor the ability to participate effectively. NHTSA recommended the use of such measures as mass mailing to all interested persons and organizations, as well as a Federal

Register notice, technical guidance by the funding body, and processing of awards as expeditiously as possible.

NHTSA also suggested that the evaluating body, which selects qualified participants for funding, be given an independent status in its deliberations. This would "protect the agency from the appearance of unfairness in selecting applicants" and lessen the possibility that funding agencies would make awards to groups with a predictable point of view. NHTSA favored retention of the evaluating body within the agency on the grounds that the separation of evaluating procedures from funding procedures would unduly complicate the rule-making process and cause unnecessary delays in processing applications.(32)

Chairman Collier of the FTC similarly supported the idea of an independent evaluating body. He suggested, however, that this authority be assigned to a body separate from the funding agency on the grounds that the separation would facilitate Congressional oversight, lend credibility to the awards, provide uniform administration of tests of financial need and pay schedules, and avoid the risk of favoritism.(33)

Current proposals for regulatory reform, S.262 and S.755, embody the notion of an independent body to determine which groups wold receive financial awards and how much they would receive.(34)

Federal experience also demonstrates the substantial administrative problems that can be associated with intervenor-funding programs. Funding determinations involve such thorny issues as the criteria for eligibility, the amount of funding, what types of proceedings are to be covered, the timing of payments, penalties for misbehavior, and judicial review of agency decisions. If only the first of these issues, eligibility, is examined, the extent of the problem is evident.

The controversial issues related to eligibility criteria center on representation of the public interest and determination of financial need. The major federal legislation dealing with these questions shows subtle and substantial variations in funding criteria. The Magnuson-Moss Act set three conditions: (1) the person or group must represent an interest which would not otherwise be adequately represented; (2) such representation must be necessary for a "fair determination"; and (3) the applicant must be financially unable to participate effectively without such compensation.

These criteria pose practical problems. Does the first criterion, for example, require the intervenor to describe his or her distinctive contribution in advance? Does the second require that the representation be indispensable to the outcome? Finally, does the third require that a petitioner demonstrate the lack of access to alternative sources of funds and furnish a full description of one's financial status?

The two Kennedy bills, to provide for intervenor funding on a governmentwide basis, contain criteria which appear to be more skillfully drafted and easier to implement. To qualify for funding, a person or group must: (1) represent an interest which could contribute substantially to a fair determination, considering the nature of the issue and the need to represent balanced interests and (2) show that one's/its economic interests in the outcome are small or that one/it lacks sufficient resources to participate effectively without the subsidy. These standards have been embodied in the regulatory reform acts proposed by the Senate Committee and the administration. When this provision is coupled with the provision for centralized administration by a single body, the administrative problems associated with funding are likely to be more readily resolved.

Both the regulatory reform proposals link intervenor funding with a weakening of procedural safeguards in regulatory proceedings. In the interests of enhancing efficiency and reducing regulatory delays, they call for the conversion of formal adjudicatory hearings into informal, legislative types of proceedings. Specifically, the proposed acts amend Section 554 of the Administrative Procedure Act so as to limit existing rights to a full adjudicatory hearing in any rate-making, rule-making, or initial licensing proceeding. Parties would have an opportunity to submit written data and arguments, to respond to written questions, and to present oral arguments on the relevant facts and questions of law contained in the written submissions. An opportunity for cross examination of witnesses would come, however, only at the conclusion of a proceeding and then only if the presiding officer were to feel the need for resolution of specific factual disputes.

Many public-interest groups believe that the move toward legislative hearings, in which reliance is placed on the preparation of a well-documented case in advance of the hearing, lends increased urgency to the call for financing of needy groups who lack their own experts. At the same time, they point out that cross examination and discovery, the traditional tools of participants at adversary hearings, are enormously valuable for testing the validity of competing arguments. To circumscribe the right to use these tools would impair the ability of hearing officers to arrive at a reasoned decision. That this is so would be particularly true in the case of complex technical issues, on which professional experts and scientists often disagree.

It is argued, moreover, that the proposed procedures would not necessarily result in saving time because presiding officers at regulatory hearings presently have the means to control discovery, cross examination, and the use of dilatory tactics by the parties. It is also noted that the distinction

between questions of fact and questions of law is so imprecise
that legal wrangles will ensue. Finally, it is suggested that
an alteration of adjudicatory procedures and the attendant loss
of procedural protections might cause appellate courts to pay
less deference to determinations made after abbreviated
procedures and to examine the evidence anew.(35)

FINDINGS

The public-hearing process was referred to initially as the
critical point for access and input of citizens at regulatory
proceedings. It is there that the significant issues of
regulatory policy are debated and resolved; and it is there
that public-interest groups particularly need help in the form
of financial and technical assistance. Many federal agencies
have apparently been willing to respond to this need, and
their responses can be interpreted as an implicit recognition on
their parts that the benefits of intervenor funding outweigh
the perceived disadvantages.

There is a very real question, however, of whether the
type of ad hoc agency-by-agency action which has been
described here will be sufficient to result in the adoption of
measures favorable to intervention by additional regulatory
industries. While it can be argued that ad hoc action may
serve each agency's needs best, there are substantial reasons
for supporting Congressional passage of a comprehensive
intervenor-funding program. It would assure intervention in
additional proceedings and relieve each agency of the need to
defend the adoption or continuation of a funding program
before its oversight committee. It would assure some minimum
level of funding in regulatory proceedings and would establish
uniform standards of eligibility and administration.

At the same time, it is important that support of
intervenor funding on a governmentwide basis not be used as
a quid pro quo for changing the rules of the regulatory
process and limiting the use of full adjudicatory procedures.
The need for intervenor funding should be judged on its own
merits, regardless of changes which may be sought in the
Administrative Procedure Act. If the move toward intervenor
funding results in a dilution of the basic protection afforded
affected parties in the regulatory process, the basic purpose
of intervention - more effective citizen participation - will not
be accomplished.

NOTES

(1)   Edgar Shor, ed., Symposium on "Public Interest Repre-
       sentation and the Federal Agencies," Public Administra-
       tion Review, XXXVII (March/April, 1977), pp. 131-54;
       Judith A. Hermanson, "Regulatory Reform by Statute:
       The Implications of the Consumer Product Safety Com-
       mission's 'Offeror System,'" Public Administration Review,
       XXXVII (March/April, 1978), pp. 205-14, respectively.
(2)   Peter H. Schuck, "Public Interest Groups and the Policy
       Process," Public Administration Review, XXXVII
       (March/April, 1977), p. 137.
(3)   Ibid.
(4)   Max D. Paglin and Edgar Shor, "Regulatory Agency
       Responses to the Development of Public Participation,"
       Public Administration Review, XXXVII (March/April,
       1977), p. 147.
(5)   Esther Peterson, the President's assistant for consumer
       affairs, is lending strong support to proposals which
       would permit departments and agencies to reimburse costs
       of citizens' participation in their proceedings. National
       Journal (August 5, 1978), p. 1241, and New York Times,
       (January 14, 1979), p. 13.
(6)   Energy Daily (August 18, 1978), p. 2, and DOE Infor-
       mation, II (Week ending October 17, 1978), p. 3.
(7)   Greene County Planning Board v. Federal Energy
       Regulatory Commission, Brief for the Federal Energy
       Regulatory Commission (FERC), on petition for a Writ of
       Certiorari to the U.S. Court of Appeals for the 2d
       Circuit, No. 77-481 (January, 1978), and the Public
       Utility Regulatory Policies Act of 1978, P.L. 95-617, Sec.
       212, respectively.
(8)   Letter from Comptroller General Elmer Staats to FTC
       Chairman Miles Kirkpatrick, August 10, 1972.
(9)   Greene County Planning Board v. Federal Power Com-
       mission, 559F. 2d 1227 (2d Cir. 1976); rev'd on
       rehearing en banc, 559F. 2d at 1237; cert. denied, 434
       U.S. 1086 (1978).
(10)   See note 7.
(11)   Letter from John M. Harmon, Assistant Attorney General
       to Phillip J. Bakes, Jr., General Counsel, CAB, and to
       Linda Heller Kamm, General Counsel, DOT, March 1,
       1978.
(12)   U.S. Chamber of Commerce v. U.S. Department of
       Agriculture, 229F. 2. 1229 (2 Cir. 19, 1978).
(13)   U.S. Congress, House, Committee on Interstate and
       Foreign Commerce, Subcommittee on Oversight and In-
       vestigations, Federal Regulation and Regulatory Reform,
       94th Cong., 2d Sess. (October 1976), pp. 481-82.

(14) U.S. Congress, Senate, Committee on Governmental Af-
      fairs,   Study on Federal Regulation: Public Participation
      in Regulatory Agency Proceedings, vol. III (July 1977),
      pp. vii and xiii, respectively.
(15) Ibid.
(16) U.S. Congress, Senate, Committee on Governmental
      Affairs,   Public Participation in Regulatory Agency
      Proceedings, vii. 94th Cong., p. 13, vol. III, July,
      1977.
(17) Ibid.
(18) Ibid., p. 20. In confirmation, Steven Ebbin and
      Raphael Kasper find that "[the administrative hearings]
      are essentially exercises in which government and in-
      dustry have tended to become allied against small groups
      of concerned, even worried, citizens. Clearly, the
      weight of influence, talent, money, power, policy and
      decision making lies with government and with industry"
      (Citizens Groups and the Nuclear Power Controversy: Use
      of Scientific and Technological Information (Cambridge:
      MIT Press, 1974), p. 251.
(19) R. D. Comfort, "Agency Assistance to Impecunious
      Intervenors," Harvard Law Review, LXXXVII (1975), p.
      1816.
(20) U.S. Congress, Senate, Committee on the Judiciary,
      Hearings, On S.2715, Public Participation in Federal
      Agency Proceedings, 94th Cong., 2d Sess., 1976, p. 86.
(21) Consolidated Edison Company (Indian Point 2), ALAB-177
      (February 26, 1974), p. 3.
(22) U.S. Congress, Senate, Committee on Governmental
      Affairs,   Public Participation in Regulatory Agency
      Proceedings, p. 114. op.
(23) See, for example, William O. Doub, Address to the
      Atomic Industrial Forum, reported in the Congressional
      Record, Senate, S.18733 (October 10, 1974), p. 22.
(24) U.S. Congress, Senate, Committee on the Judiciary,
      Hearings on S.2715, 1976, pp. 17-18. On this point, see
      also D. Stephen Cupps, "Emerging Problems of Citizen
      Participation," Public Administration Review, XXXVII
      (September/October, 1977), p. 482.
(25) Tersh Boasberg et al., Policy Issues Raised by Inter-
      venor Requests for Financial Assistance in NRC
      Proceedings, Report to the Nuclear Regulatory Com-
      mission (July 18, 1975), pp. 120-23. See also Cupps,
      Public Administration Review, XXXVII (September/Oc-
      tober, 1977), p. 480.
(26) U.S. Congress, Senate, Senate Report 94-863, 94th
      Cong., 2d Sess. (1976), p. 52.
(27) "Funding Public Participation in Regulatory Pro-
      ceedings," Regulation (March/April, 1978), p. 10.

(28) U.S. Congress, Senate, testimony before the Senate Committee on the Judiciary on S.270, Public Participation in Federal Agency Proceedings Act of 1977 (February 3, 1977), pp. 1 and 6.
(29) FTC Press Release, "FTC Public Participation Program" (February 1, 1979).
(30) National Highway Traffic Safety Administration, "Department of Transportation's Demonstration Program to Provide Financial Assistance to Participants in Administrative Proceedings" (June 14, 1977), p. 3.
(31) Ibid., 16.
(32) Ibid., 18.
(33) U.S. Congress, Senate, Testimony before the Senate Committee on the Judiciary on S.270, 1977, pp. 9-12.
(34) See, for example, David Cohen, "Citizen Participation in Government," paper presented at a meeting cosponsored by the Aspen Institute for Humanistic Studies and Common Cause (March 8, 1979), pp. 12-15.
(35) See, for example, Institute for Public Representation, National Resources Defense Council and Congress Watch, "Comments on Proposed Administrative Procedure Reform Legislation" (January 12, 1979), letter to Ms. Judy Areen, Office of Management and Budget, January 23, 1979; and "Comments on Draft Regulatory Reform Act," February 12, 1979.

6 Ambiguity as a Source of Political Efficacy: The Contradictions of the German Antinuclear Movement*

Michael Pollak

The discussion of the ecology movement among German political scientists focuses on questions about the legitimacy of the citizens' initiatives that are its main units of organization.(1) Are these widespread citizens' initiatives an illegal expression of political interests, since mediation between government and people is an activity that the German constitution explicitly reserves for political parties?(2) Are these initiatives a new vehicle for Communist subversion? The questions determine the answers: Conservative authors, often having legal backgrounds, emphasize the potential dangers for the system of representative democracy;(3) liberal authors in favor of the initiatives stress their stabilizing effect by arguing that they allow the expression of grass-roots concerns and should be taken into account in policy making.(4) The radical left is split in its interpretation of the new phenomenon: some argue, in a manner analogous to that of the conservative tradition, that the citizen initiatives are but the first step of a revolutionary overthrow of the ruling class;(5) others, having views similar to the liberal line, argue that the citizens' initiatives, a typical middle-class phenomenon, will be co-opted by the administration through the development of additional participatory channels. Thus, in the long run, it is argued, they will strengthen the legitimacy of the system.(6)

Each of these interpretations is motivated by political sympathy or antipathy toward the citizens' initiatives. The political scientists' fixation on legal criteria and formal organizations prevents them from recognizing the citizens'

*This article was written as part of a research project funded by the German Marshall Fund.

70

initiatives for what they are - the expression of a social movement. For the activists on the other hand, the problems of legitimacy and organization in the traditional political sense do not exist. "The new groupings call themselves a movement and it does not matter to them whether they are accepted as a movement by the social sciences; they are active as a movement, are accepted by the public as a movement, and are remembered as a movement after their end."(7)

The antinuclear movement had its roots in the rapid economic and social changes of the postwar period; it appeals in particular to those segments of the population most affected by these changes. The heterogeneity of its potential constituency determines the diversity of its organizational forms and of its arguments. The movement has to maintain a fragile balance between the tactics it uses to influence administrative decision making and those it uses in extraparliamentary actions. It must both prove its effectiveness and keep its social base mobilized. Therefore, the apparent contradictions of the ecology movement and the ambiguity of its tactics are less an indication of its inability to achieve higher levels of organization than they are sources of its efficacy.

THE SOCIAL ROOTS OF THE MOVEMENT

The historical analysis of social conflicts(8) and of marginal social movements(9) suggests that they arise from important and relatively rapid changes in economic and social structure that lead to conflict among the social groups or classes that are favored and threatened by these changes. Information about the past cannot directly explain the present; nevertheless, the passage of time provides a removed perspective, independent of the ongoing debate about nuclear energy, that is necessary for the formulation of hypotheses concerning the origin and the structure of the antinuclear movement.

German economic growth after 1945 was extremely rapid compared to that in Germany's past and that of its neighbors.

Table 6.1: German Economic Growth 1870-1970
(Average BNP growth rate in %)

1870-1913	2.9%	German Reich
1913-1950	1.2%	German Reich
1950-1960	8.5%	Federal Republic
1960-1970	4.8%	Federal Republic

Source: OECD, Statistics, 1974.

Germany's growth rate in the 1950s (8.5 percent) was twice as high as that of France. The reconstruction of the country and the immigration of around 19 million refugees from the eastern parts of the Reich account for part of this growth, which was accompanied by rapid industrial concentration and urbanization. At the same time, the socioprofessional composition of the population changed drastically: Agricultural employment dropped from 22 percent in 1950 to 7 percent in 1975; manufacturing and industrial employment increased from slightly more than 40 percent in 1945 to 48 percent in 1961 and subsequently stabilized and then decreased slowly to around 42 percent in the late 1970s. The tertiary sector has increased from 33 percent in 1950 to 47 percent in 1975, with a particularly marked increase in employment in skilled office and managerial work.(10) Another important change has been the increase of university education, which more than doubled in the 1960s.(11)

Economic expansion brought with it a corresponding ideology: a modernistic faith in progress which is identified with an urban life-style and is measured by an increase in available income and material goods. The recession of 1976, however, called into question the dream of an unlimited linear economic growth. It also showed that despite the built-in controls and regulations of economic policy, capitalist development is still subject to cyclical crises. The crisis of the world monetary system since the end of the 1960s and the oil crisis of 1973 have led to stagnation and recession and to direct questioning of the ideology of unlimited growth. The increasing intensity of social conflicts in Germany since the mid-1960s may be interpreted as an emergence of the potential for conflict that accumulated during previous years, when political consensus, a result of the war catastrophe, and the necessity of reconstruction kept open conflict to a minimum.

THE EMERGENCE OF THE ANTINUCLEAR MOVEMENT

The conflicts that began to develop in the late 1960s arose not only over the traditional issues of wages and working conditions, but also out of dissatisfaction with the living conditions. Issues such as transportation, urban planning, and nursery schools moved people to organize "citizens' initiatives." The quality of the modern urban life-style was less and less taken for granted. The quality of the natural environment outside of the polluted urban centers became of increasing concern. Dissatisfaction with living conditions and the rise of expectations about leisure time created a new sensitivity among groups increasingly open to the arguments of the ecology movement.

Very large initiatives were triggered off in major cities by substantial increases in public transportation fares, the first being the "Rote-Punkt-Aktion" in Hannover in 1969, often referred to as the start of a citizens'-initiative wave. In Frankfurt between 1970 and 1973, urban renewal was resisted by squatting in houses and by frequently violent demonstrations against the demolition of entire districts for the purpose of office construction and land speculation.

Surveys of the citizens' initiatives indicate that their main activities focus on sociocultural and environmental problems. A survey in Bavaria in 1972 found that 43 percent of the initiatives were concerned with the environment (including aspects of nuclear power) and that 42 percent were concerned with sociocultural matters such as nurseries, youth clubs, community facilities, and protection of a common heritage. Another survey carried out in the industrial center of the Ruhr provided comparable results: 45 percent of the initiatives were organized around environmental issues and 31 percent around sociocultural matters. A survey conducted in Berlin gave appreciably different results: 40 percent of the initiatives concerned housing and urban development problems.(12)

In Germany as a whole, the categories of issues treated by the initiatives can be divided as follows: environment, 16.9 percent; transportation, 11.8 percent; kindergartens and sports facilities, 15.8 percent; schools, 8.1 percent; urban development, 8 percent; marginal groups, 7.1 percent; cultural life and heritage, 5.7 percent; youth problems, 4.9 percent; community facilities, 3.9 percent; urban sanitation, 3.6 percent; and cultural activities, 3.3 percent.(13)

The weak organization of the citizens'-initiative groups is often seen as their main characteristic. Local initiatives often exist no longer than a year, and success in achieving their goals brings their end. But this is less the case for the initiatives in the field of environment. Their local struggles often take a long time, and the large implications of most decisions affecting the environment have resulted in regional and national coordination of groups through the Bundesverband Burgerinitiativen Umweltschutz (BBU). Created in 1972, this umbrella organization serves as a communications center, maintains contact with experts willing to cooperate, gives tactical advice, lobbies on environmental issues in Bonn, and provides a connection to the European Bureau of the Environment in Brussels, which coordinates the lobbying efforts of the environmental organizations in the EEC-Commission. In early 1977, surveys estimated the existence of some 50,000 initiatives, which all together were estimated to have as many members as all political parties (around 1.5 million).(14)

One cannot interpret these numbers too literally, but they unquestionably represent an important political phenomenon.

Further empirical investigations suggest that these large numbers in fact indicate what portion of the population can be mobilized for specific actions. The "hard core" of individual citizens' initiatives usually contains no more than between 10 and 30 members who meet regularly and devote an important amount of their time preparing for actions, compiling technical dossiers, meeting with bureaucrats, etc.(15) Often these activists are at the same time members of a party or other influential social organizations which help them to muster external support.(16)

Even the traditional and rather apolitical organizations for the conservation of nature were politicized by the growth of public interest in ecological issues. Under pressure from the most active parts of their constituency, most of them support the objectives of environmental citizens' initiatives and evaluate their actions as a positive contribution to the environmental policy process.(17)

It was the issue of nuclear power that expanded concern for the environment to dissent on a national scale. Reviving the tradition of the extraparliamentary opposition of the 1960s, several thousand people mobilized in 1977 for demonstrations at plant sites.

SOCIAL HETEROGENEITY AND FLEXIBLE ORGANIZATION

There is more potential support for ecological and, in particular, antinuclear initiatives than that which comes from those directly concerned about specific pollution projects.(18) The subject of nuclear power has come to involve a set of preoccupations and anxieties about the character of rapid technological and social change: There is concern about the effect of technological change on the social and economic structure, the industrialization of rural areas, the concentration of economic activities, the centralization of decision making, and the incremental tendencies toward a tightening of police control. Critics talk less of nuclear energy than of a "nuclear society."

Those attracted by the ecological and antinuclear movements are socially heterogeneous because of the broad impact of recent structural and economic changes. Surveys indicate that there is an overrepresentation of the educated middle classes and an effective mobilization of farmers when they are directly affected by a technological change. A detailed analysis reveals the following characteristics of the citizens' initiatives:

First, there is a clear correlation between the aim of an initiative and the social characteristics of its members. For example, a citizens' initiative arising in reaction to an urban development measure in a district with a homogeneous population will be characterized by the same homogeneity. It may be expected that the social breakdown of citizens' initiatives involving regional or citywide problems will largely correspond to that prevailing in the city or region. But in general, the citizens' initiatives include relatively few workers and a high proportion of middle-class members, who usually have liberal and intellectual professions.(19)

The figures obtained in surveys of initiatives contain a systematic bias: mostly gathered in urban areas, they do not include the agricultural population. Case studies have shown, especially in the nuclear case, that agricultural populations are difficult to mobilize in response to general political issues but are rapidly and easily mobilized in a local struggle once they perceive a threat to economic conditions.(20) They are indeed easy to mobilize when major technological projects threaten to affect the environment, the climate, and, indirectly, agricultural production. Further empirical evidence suggests that surveys of citizens' initiatives give only a limited picture of the capacity of environmental and, in particular, nuclear issues for inspiring mobilization. According to opinion polls, some two million Germans took part in one or more initiatives in 1975 and 1976. The scale of this commitment to political action is clear, for the total membership of the political parties is 1.8 million. Only 12 percent of the population would consider joining a political party, but 34 percent would participate in a citizens' initiative.(21) If their personal interests were directly involved, 60 percent of the population would participate in an initiative. In 1977, the BBU claimed to cover 900 groups, which together have more than 200,000 members.

All these figures indicate that the popular support for the environmental movement and for its most active and politicized part, the antinuclear movement, extends far beyond that of the exclusive middle-class permanent activists. Its main support comes from the rural population and from the new educated middle classes. The workers are significantly less well represented.

The nuclear conflict has united peripheral classes. Referring to this social diversity, some sympathizers have argued that the movement cuts across all parts of society and represents the common interest; critics, in contrast, have emphasized its middle-class character. However, the cautious statements coming from the labor movement and the evolution of a union position based on almost exclusively economic considerations call for a different interpretation. Capital and labor are apparently united in favor of promoting nuclear energy by a short-term perception of their class interests. Thus, the nuclear debate can be analyzed as a class conflict, dominated by those groups that have been most affected by recent structural changes.

But the peripheral classes and portions of classes united by a common antinuclear position have diverging interests in almost all other dimensions. For decades, the farmers were relatively marginal politically, and their political activity was limited to a powerful direct representation of their interests within the conservative parties. Even though their view on the nuclear issue is opposed to the Christian Democrats' (CDU/CSU) endorsement of nuclear energy, these traditional ties are nevertheless significant. The educated modern middle classes and, especially, the young generation influenced by the student movement of the 1960s link their concern about nuclear energy with broader objectives for societal change. They are politically rather to the left, and they are typically motivated by an enlightened humanism. They attempt to maintain open communication with the governmental Social Democratic (SPD) and Liberal (FDP) parties and with the labor unions. In an interview, the former chairman of the BBU, Hans Helmut Wustenhagen, said:(22)

> Everything now depends on a pact with the labor unions. If we do obtain such a pact, we are sure to win. If we do not obtain it, then one must be very pessimistic.

This diversity of interests shapes the context in which the antinuclear movement must maneuver if it is to keep its constituency together. For its rather conservative members, it must emphasize the legitimacy of its organization, argumentation, and strategy with respect to the constitutional political order. For the more progressive activists from a radical tradition, it must emphasize the potential changes in the system that it might eventually bring about. This maneuvering determines the organization of the movement. It has to be sufficiently well-organized so that its spokesmen can support their lobbying efforts by documenting the size of the group, but the organization has to be flexible enough to prevent internal ideological clashes. A loose organization is not a contradiction of political success, but is rather a condition of it. When the leader of the BBU speculates about the possibility of challenging the liberal vote in elections(23) and at the same time argues that the citizens' initiatives are in no way a new political party but rather a complementary element meant to improve communication between government and the citizenry,(24) he is satisfying the concerns of several types of constituents. The BBU presents itself as the most important mass-movement pressure group,(25) at the same time that it claims to be a model of direct democracy, thereby implying the absence of a structured formal organization.(26) To characterize the citizens' initiatives as unorganized is certainly misleading. While not organized in a hierarchical manner, with clear-cut lines of command, the organization can best be described as a tight social network of people sharing strong common interests and values. They devote a large proportion of their time to the common cause, meet regularly, have a well-functioning system of communication through regular publications,(27) and maintain contact with experts ready to collaborate in administrative or legal proceedings. Without a formal hierarchy, there exists a leadership arising from the exigencies of an efficient defense of the cause. Most of those informal leaders are good public speakers and are able to establish useful links with influential social organizations. At the regional and national level, the required formation of legally recognized voluntary associations empowered to speak in the name of their constituency and to deal as interest associations with the bureaucracy also forced a structuring of the organization and the formation of a national leadership. When the media focuses attention on the leadership, it further reinforces the tendency toward hierarchical structure. The very process of creating a formal leadership further increases internal conflicts and tensions, which are best illustrated by the formation of electoral groupings in 1978 (see below). In sum, the need to unify a very heterogeneous constituency forces the antinuclear movement to maintain the greatest possible flexibility as well as to develop the minimum formal structure necessary to influence the policy process.

APOCALYPTIC IMAGERY AND TECHNICAL EXPERTISE

The ambiguities in the social composition and organization of the antinuclear movement are reflected in its arguments. Addressing people deeply affected by the larger socioeconomic crisis of the last few years, the activists tend at first to stress the disastrous potential consequences of this crisis. Their apocalyptic style helps to unify heterogeneous interests. Their arguments are largely reactive. Ecological problems, particularly nuclear risks, are presented as the most important global issues faced by mankind today. This humanistic reasoning has sensitized a broad population.

In the early 1970s, exploitation of scarce natural resources was attacked as irresponsible and disastrous for the future.(28)

The most convincing emotional argument for involvement in the antinuclear movement is the possibility of nuclear catastrophe. One finds again and again in antinuclear pamphlets a set of powerful images of death and war. Nuclear power plants are presented as "quasiweapons" and are said to be threats not only because of the possibility of a major accident, but also because of the long term effects of

radiation, an "invisible slowly operating death of the society."
In the visual presentations of antinuclear literature, these
images have a powerful impact; nuclear forces are often
represented as skeletons, which are contrasted with the symbol
of a smiling sun that represents the antinuclear movement.

The nuclear imagery is inseparably linked to Hiroshima
and Nagasaki. But this imagery is subtly extended to suggest
that in a nuclear society there is a permanent civil war.(29)
The activists oppose nuclear power on the grounds that it
might lead to reinforcement of social control and police
repression. They also point out the fragility of a highly
technological society, in which a small, well-planned act of
sabotage or terrorism can lead to unforeseeable consequences.

Such dramatization lends urgency to the nuclear issue and
forces people to take a definite position for or against it. But
dramatization can only succeed if the arguments used
correspond to reality. Activists use documents on occasional
accidents in power plants to counter the official claim that
nuclear power is the safest of all energy sources, and they
suggest that a highly improbable accident could happen one
day. Illegal supervision of individuals such as that in the
Traube case(30) nourishes fears of the advent of a police
state. The violence of the clashes between demonstrators and
police forces is referred to in the media in a way that
suggests that there is already a state of civil war.(31)

The apocalyptic imagery of the antinuclear activists has
brought them a reputation as reactive, negative, and above
all, incapable of proposing alternatives. Actually, the societal
alternatives proposed by the most politicized groups begin from
a criticism of the existing socioeconomic order. All claim that
the nuclear option fails to reflect a democratic consensus and
that it was imposed by a powerful industrial
scientific-government complex. The antinuclear activists
identify this new power elite as their main enemy. But they
differ about what strategies should be employed to oppose this
establishment, partly as a result of the emphasis accorded to
different aspects of the socioeconomic analysis. At one
extreme, the analysis may lead to revolutionary interpretations
that revise anarcho-syndicalist traditions of social organization
based on small self-regulating units. A similar analysis leads
to the idea of a utopia of "conviviality," a society freed from
the agressions engendered by competition and the search for
material goods. The success of Ivan Illich's books indicates
the power of this ideology.(32)

The emphasis on economic analysis has also resulted in
more classical Marxist proposals; the centralist tradition of
major labor movement organizations is often translated into
proposals for tighter state regulations implying the
growth of environmental bureaucracies in the government.
The ecologists fighting for decentralized solutions attack this

coming "ecotechnocracy" as being almost as dangerous for civil freedom as the "nuclear technocracy."

Yet other groups believe in the possibility of slow, step-by-step reforms. They propose to copy for the purpose of environmental policy the model provided by Social-partnershaft in economic policy. They say that industry, government, and the representatives of environmental associations and citizens' initiatives should meet regularly to work out pragmatic proposals to solve the ecological crisis. Indeed, the discussion forum "Arbeisgemeinschaft fur Umweltfragen" was intended to fulfill this role. This association, created in 1972, has brought together antagonistic social actors. But the environmental group representatives have successfully prevented the transformation of the informal debate on general issues into specific policy discussions which might serve to legitimate governmental policies.

Those groups emphasizing the apocalyptic visions of the coming nuclear society and ecological collapse sometimes generate highly traditional ideologies. In the German context they often have a nationalist flavor and contain almost racist elements. But these groups represent only a margin of the whole movement. Their names frequently indicate their ideological orientation: Weltbund zum Schutz des Lebens (World Association for the Protection of Life), Gesellschaft fur Erbgesundheitspflege (Association for the Cultivation of Hereditary Health). Some groups linked to the national-liberal sport association Turnerbund share the same ideology. Leftist critics call these groups the "eco-fascists."(33)

Apocalyptic visions are also typical of various marginal sects and counterculture groups of the younger generation. Far Eastern religious groups, in particular the Taoists, with their holistic character, oppose the rational, analytical Western philosophy which, by dividing up reality, has lost the sense of organic relations. In these counterculture groups the ecological issues are often mixed with various other beliefs, e.g., vegetarianism, astrology, etc.

To a certain extent all groups include in their reasoning some utopian reference to a golden age of still-innocent nature. But while apocalyptic approaches exploit widespread dissatisfaction with the prevailing materialist values, more analytic and political approaches dominate the antinuclear movement. This gives the ecological and antinuclear movement a two-sided, regressive-progressive character. The construction of models for a future society out of idyllic images of the past converges in the movement with general moods of the 1970s - nostalgia and fatigue from the rhythm of too rapid change.

Beyond the ideological features that provide mobilizing force, the antinuclear movement needs technical expertise to advance its cause. Efforts to influence governmental decisions through lobbying or complaints in administrative courts can be effective only if backed by technical resources. And the antinuclear movement has managed to find many experts. The controversy on nuclear energy is characterized by the presence of expertise on both sides in almost all involved areas and disciplines. This phenomenon indicates two things. First, in a highly technological society, the credibility of a social movement depends on its ability to invoke expert knowledge. Therefore, access to expertise as a political resource is a condition of political influence. Second, the conflicts among the experts themselves concerning nuclear safety preclude all attempts to narrow down the nuclear issue to its technical aspects.

TACTICAL OSCILLATIONS

In a highly variegated and even contradictory movement, tactics are often incoherent and subject to sudden changes. Nevertheless, there have been three distinct phases of the antinuclear movement. The first phase consisted of local actions and consciousness raising. During this phase, many activists believed that argument alone could bring about policy changes. Second came a phase of mass mobilization marked by violence and major confrontations with the police. Third was a search for balance in which the movement sought to adapt while retaining its independence.

The first important actions were carried out at Wyhl, in the wine-growing region of the Lower Rhine.(34) The wine growers were concerned about the possible effects of nuclear construction on the climate. The first public hearing of the licensing procedure, in 1973, revealed the hostility of the population. But the Christian Democratic government of the Land, convinced that the protest resulted more from Communist subversion than from local concerns, ignored the protest. The ecologists therefore used different means to stop construction: peaceful demonstrations, petitions, delegations to the Land government, and court action. The support of the citizens' initiatives by eminent scientists and national media coverage both helped to publicize the antinuclear arguments. Finally, in 1977, after a hearing of government experts, representatives of the electricity companies, and representatives of the citizen initiatives, the administrative court prohibited construction.

This court decision, based on only one of the technical points in a long list presented by the ecologists, was exploited as proof of the justification of the antinuclear position. Meanwhile, the debate turned into a confrontation between two moral positions, leaving no space for negotiations. Observers

spoke about a "modern religious war" between diametrically
opposed beliefs about the future. Proponents of nuclear power
argued that only nuclear energy could meet world energy
needs, while opponents insisted that nuclear power would
destroy mankind. Each side felt the issue was survival.(35)
When the antinuclear activists decided in 1977 to occupy sites
at Brokdorf and Grohnde, violent clashes were the inevitable
result. The antinuclear position was adamant. Convinced of
the truth of their position and of their moral superiority, the
leading antinuclear activists overestimated their capacity and
made major tactical mistakes. In social reality, it is power,
not the truth or morality of an argument, that decides public
policy. In the absence of a revolutionary situation, a direct
confrontation with government, which holds a monopoly of legal
and physical strength, could lead only to failure. When the
BBU announced after the mass demonstration at Kalkar that it
no longer considered such spectacular actions as the main
tactical instrument, observers predicted the death of the
antinuclear movement.

This perceived end was only a period of major tactical
reorientation, meant to widen the scope of negotiations with
decision makers. In this process of adaptation to the political
context, the antinuclear movement oscillates between
independence and integration into the political system, which is
best illustrated by the 1978 participation in regional
elections.(36)

When a social movement tries to turn itself into a party
organization, internal conflicts arise and it risks losing most of
its supporters. Only in Lower Saxony, where the ecologists
were united by the struggle against the reprocessing and
waste disposal plant in Gorleben, could they present a common
platform. In Hamburg, three ecological parties competed: a
conservative "green list"; an old, "environmentalized" splinter
party; and the leftist, antiauthoritarian "colored list." In
Hessen the ecologists ranged on a continuum from those in the
respectable, conservative "Action Future," created by the
former CDU spokesman for environmental problems Gruhl, to
the spontaneous counterculture radicals centered around the
hero of May 1968, Daniel Cohn-Bendit.

But despite these organizational schisms, the elections
have shown that the antinuclear movement is alive and could,
under changed conditions, remobilize its support. In Hamburg
and Lower Saxony the vote of the ecologists equaled the liberal
vote and eliminated the FDP from the regional parliaments. In
Hamburg the "colored list" united on its radical platform
ecologists, women's liberation supporters, prisoners,
homosexuals, and opposers of the Berufsverbote. With almost
25 percent of the vote it was second only to the SPD in
dominating the 18-to-25 age group.(37) Only in Hessen,
where the split among the ecologists was the deepest and

where the elections were dominated by national concerns, was electoral participation a complete failure for the movement.

These examples lead to the conclusion that the antinuclear movement and its heterogeneous constituency must find their way by relying on various tactical maneuvers from both outside and inside the official decision-making procedures. But in the process of adaptation, it must avoid full integration into the political system. It simply cannot copy the organizational models of typical political life. To maintain unity among its ideologically diverging components and to survive as a social movement, it must search for a flexible balance of spontaneous tactics and structured organization. Ambiguity is therefore not a weakening factor, but is rather its main source of political efficacy.

NOTES

(1)   The eminent political science journal Zietschrift fur Parlamentsfragen has devoted a special issue to this theme. See vol. 1, March 1978. In the last few years more than 300 books and articles have been published on the citizens' initiatives, most centering around the legitimacy theme. See the bibliography put together by W. Welz in: B. Guggenberger, V. Kempf, eds., Burger-initiativen und Reprasentatives System, WDV, Opladen, 1978, pp. 375-380.

(2)   L. J. Edinger, Politics in Germany (Boston: Little, Brown, 1968), p. 267.

(3)   Schmidt, Organisierte Einwirkungen auf die Verwaltung, in VVDSTL, Bd. 33, 1975. A. Hartisch, Verfassungs-rechtliches Leistungsprinzip und Partizipationsverbot im Verwaltungsverfahren, (Berlin, 1975).

(4)   P. C. Mayer-Tasch, Die Burgerinitiativbewegung (Rein-bek: Rororo, 1976). U. Thaysen, "Burgerinitiativen, Parlamente und Parteien in der BRD. Eine Zwischen-bilanz," in Zeitschrift fur Parlamentsfragen, op. cit., p. 12. H. Zillessen, "'Dialog mit dem Burger' oder Beteiligung des Burgers," in SPD Forum, Energie, Beschaftigung, Lebensqualitat, Koln, 1967.

(5)   This argument is not present in the scientific discussion. It prevails in some Maoist circles.

(6)   C. Offe, Strukturprobleme des Kapitalistisschen Staates (Frankfurt: Suhrkamp, 1972), pp. 153 ff. H. Fassbinder, "Burgerinitiativen und Planungsbeteiligung im Kontext Kapitalistischer Regionalpolitik," in Kursbuch 27 (Berlin, 1972), pp. 68 ff.

(7)   O. Rammstedt, Soziale Bewegung (Frankfurt: Suhr-kamp, 1978), p. 28.

(8) C. Tilly, et al., The Rebellious Century, 1830-1930 (Cambridge: Harvard University Press, 1975), p. 97.

(9) See Hobsbawm, Sozialrebellen, Archaische Sozialbewegungen im 19 und 20 Jahrhundert, Neuwied, Luchterhand, 1962. G. Botz, G. Brandstetter, M. Pollak, Im Schatten der Arbeiterbewegung (Wien: Europa, 1977).

(10) D. Menyesch, H. Unterwedde, "Wirtschaftliche und Soziale Strukturen in der Bundesrepublik und in Frankreich," in R. Picht, ed., Deutschland, Frankreich, Europa (Munchen: Piper, 1978), p. 53.

(11) OECD, Development of Higher Education 1950-1967. Statistical Survey, Paris, 1970.

(12) Bayerisches Staatsministerium des Inneren, Burgerinitiativen in Bayern, Munchen, 1973. (Bestandsaufnahme Az I B 1-3000-72/1) B. Borsdorf-Ruhl, Burgerinitiativen im Ruhrgebiet, Essen, 1973.

(13) P. von Kondolitsch, "Gemeindeverwaltungen und Burgerinitiativen," in Archiv fur Kommunalwissenschaften, XIV (1975), p. 264.

(14) U. Thaysen, op. cit., p. 90.

(15) B. Borsdorf-Ruhl, op. cit., pp. 78 ff.

(16) One can give the leaders of the BBU as examples. Among the first 4 chairmen, one finds two high officials of the Protestant church playing an eminent role in its adult-education system, one member of the FDP and one member of the SPD.

(17) This is the result of a survey including the major national and regional associations for nature conservation. Survey conducted as part of a research project on the French and German antinuclear movement at STS Program, Cornell University, unpublished.

(18) R. Burger, "'Lebensqualitat' und Warenproduktion," in Wirtschaft und Gesellschaft 4 (1975), pp. 17 ff.

(19) The following results were obtained in a survey carried out in Berlin: 47% liberal professions, 37% teachers, 8% workers.

(20) Battelle Institut, Burgerinitiativen im Bereich von Kernkraftwerken (Bonn, 1975), compares a site in an urban area, Ludwigshaven, and in a rural area, Wyhl.

(21) Emnid-Information (Nov. 11-12, 1973), p. 7.

(22) Interview in Konkret, 4 (1977), p. 23.

(23) H.G. Schumacher, presently president of the BBU, indicated this possibility. Wirtschaftswoche, 16 (April 7, 1977).

(24) See the contribution of H.G. Schumacher in Arbeitsgemeinschaft fur Umweltfragen, Atomforum-1977 (Bonn, 1977), pp. 21 ff.

(25) U. Thaysen, op. cit., p. 90.

(26) H. Zillessen, "Energiepolitik und Burgerinitiativen," in K. Oeser, H. Zillessen, Kernenergie, Mensch, Umwelt, Wissenschaft und Politik, Koln, p. 104.

(27) B. Borsdorf-Ruhl, op. cit., pp. 78 ff. U. Thaysen,
     op. cit., p. 96.
(28) The German translation of the "Limits of Growth" report
     commissioned by the Club of Rome was the start for an
     avalanche of publications, the most popular being a book
     published by the former CDU environmental spokesman H.
     Gruhl, Ein Planet Wird Geplundert (Econ, Dusseldorf,
     1973).
(29) This is one of the main themes of the best seller R.
     Jungk, Der Atomstaat (Kindler, Munchen, 1977).
(30) Klaus Traube, manager of the nuclear firm Interatom was
     suspected to have contacts with terrorists. The German
     FBI illegally observed him and installed microphones in
     his house. Warned by the FBI, Interatom fired him.
     After publication of this affair by Der Spiegel, 10, 11,
     and 12, 1976, politicians tried to play it down.
(31) The clashes between demonstrators and the police were
     widely publicized by television and newspaper coverage.
     For a series of photos, see U. Herms, Brokdorfer
     Kriegsfibel (Hamburg: Welt Verlag, 1977), p. 212.
(32) The concept of "conviviality" proposed by Illich in order
     to characterize a new societal organization is very often
     used to describe the human qualities of the relations
     among antinuclear activists as opposed to the rigidity of
     the pronuclear forces, e.g., R. Jungk, op. cit., pp. 201
     ff.
(33) H. M. Enzenkerger, "Zur Kritik der Politischen Oko-
     logie," in Kursbuch, 33, 1973. Kommunistischer Bund,
     Antifaschistischer Steckbrief No. 3, (Hamburg: Verlag
     Arbeiterkampf, 1976.)
(34) H. H. Wustenhagen, Burger Gegen Kernkraftwerke,
     Wyhl - Der Anfang?, Rororo, Reinbek, 1975. N. Gladitz,
     Lieber Heute Aktiv als Morgen Radioaktiv, (Berlin:
     Wagenbach, 1976.)
(35) This is the formulation of the former Minister of Science
     and Technology H. Matthofer in: Der Spiegel, 14 (1977),
     p. 48.
(36) See the internal discussion of the BBU in its central
     newsletter, BBU-Aktuell, 3, 1978.
(37) Der Spiegel, 24 (1978), p. 32.

III

Education Policy

7 Education as Loosely Coupled Systems in West Germany and the United States

Maurice A. Garnier

A number of critics in Europe and the United States see education and bureaucracy as mutually incompatible (e.g., Carnoy, 1975; Baudelot and Establet, 1971). When the bureaucratic nature of educational systems is acknowledged, it is usually to decry its evils. Implicit in many radical criticisms of education is the desire to do away with bureaucracies altogether.

While much decried, educational bureaucracies have been studied little in Europe and in the United States. This neglect of educational bureaucracies means that we do not know whether the principles of organizational structure or of organizational functioning operate in educational bureaucracies. Yet educational bureaucracies must be understood before they can be changed.

A number of social characteristics make it necessary for education to be run bureaucratically and such a system of organization can have positive consequences.

SOURCES OF BUREAUCRATIZATION IN EDUCATION

The first important observation one must make about education is that it is a state responsibility. It is curious that such an obvious fact is usually not mentioned in studies of educational bureaucracies. There are several consequences of this simple fact.

The first one is that political units differ greatly in size. If the relevant educational unit is the state, as in Germany and the United States, then we will find a unit like California and another like Delaware. In Germany, we will find Hamburg and Nordrhein-Westfalen. If traditions mandate that education

be administered at the local level, then we will find units like
Los Angeles or small towns.

This definition of the unit has important consequences
because size has been shown to be one of the most important
determinants of organizational structures (Blau and
Schoenherr, 1972). Increased size usually leads to economies
of scale, so that the greater the size, the lower the
administrative ratio (Blau and Schoenherr, 1972; Hendershot
and James, 1972; Heyerbrand, 1973). Put in a practical way,
large educational bureaucracies should be able to provide
educational services at a lower cost than small units.
Alternatively, large systems have the option of funding special
programs or research with the savings thus realized. There is
also evidence that large school districts enjoy a distinct
advantage over small ones. I should note that the exact nature
of this relationship between size and administrative ratios is
not known in the case of educational organizations. What is
known is that education uses few administrators: the State of
California ran its schools with 981 persons in 1971-72 and with
9,679 principals and supervisors of instruction for the whole
state. The total for California, including maintenance,
transportation, clerical personnel, etc. was 108,000 for a state
with a population of 18 million or a total average daily
attendance of 4,453,000 for 1971-72 (National Center for
Education Statistics, 1975).

Thus, the sheer size of the relevant unit will, if
organization theory applies to schools, determine the
organizational structure which will administer education. More
important perhaps is that size determines other aspects of
organizational structure. Size can also increase centralization
of decision making under some circumstances. This particular
relationship is, in reality, indirect because size increases
specialization (Jeydebrand, 1973). This specialization leads to
the necessity for coordination, i.e., the many units which
compose a large organization need to be coordinated and one
possible solution to coordination often involves centralization of
decision making. In a large organization, the activities of
each division affect the operations of many others and,
therefore, the parochial point of view which necessarily
prevails in each subunit must be reconciled with the overall
interests of the entire organization. Decisions can be made at
a high level within the organization or, alternatively, rules can
be established by high-level officials so that the decisions
made within subunits do not jeopardize other units. What goes
on within the mathematics department from carrying out its obligations. What
goes on in secondary schools within a school district cannot
jeopardize what goes on in elementary schools, etc.
Thus, typically, school districts have a director of secondary education and a director of elementary education whose

activities are coordinated hierarchically by the superintendent of schools. Even in school systems which allow their subordinates considerable autonomy, as in Britain, such coordination always takes place. Hierarchical coordination, however, constitutes only one of the methods which can be used; other methods do exist.

Increased size will usually result in specialization of tasks which, in turn, will generate centralization of decision making. It is, therefore, important to remember that students of educational bureaucracies must take into account the fact that the size of the units they will study is given to them. Once the size of the political unit has been determined through the political process, then the work of the student of bureaucracy may start.

In addition to determining the geographical unit which will constitute a "system," politicians tell educators who in fact may or may not be educated. Actually, the sheer size of the cohort is usually not under the control of politicians or educators. Birth rates and migrations determine the number of children who will enter schools. Thus, school districts grow rapidly or slowly lose population. Increase or decrease in population will also affect the size of schools, the number of schools, and, eventually, the entire administrative apparatus of the school district. Growth in population resulting from demographic increases has been shown to alter administrative ratios in the United States, and it is likely that such efforts could be demonstrated in other settings as well (Hendershot, et al., 1972).

While demographic changes are not usually within the control of politicians or educators, other kinds of numerical changes are. As a result of perceived economic needs and an increased demand for educational opportunities, the definition of who qualifies for school has been altered in all industrialized countries. If citizens believe that kindergarten is necessary and if the state responds to that request for increased services, then the number of kindergartens will increase. The same applies to secondary education which has experienced huge increases in virtually all industrialized countries. The creation of new secondary schools affects teachers' colleges, affects budgetary considerations and, in all likelihood, affects the entire system. Experienced teachers will need to receive additional training so that they might qualify as heads of the new schools. Assignment policies or recruitment policies will need to be implemented, the activities of secondary schools will need to be coordinated and the process of differentiation will take place. If the increased population is accommodated within the existing schools, then these schools will increase in size and new services will be required: health, vocational counseling, etc. At any rate, the increased number of mathematics teachers, for example, will

result in the creation of heads of departments or coordinators
for mathematics. Assistant principals will have to coordinate
their activities and scheduling will become more complex.
Principals will need additional training in accounting and other
administrative skills, and thus, some additional professional
training will be developed for them. Soon, a traditional,
stable system has become highly differentiated and the need
for coordination arises. Typically, such coordination will take
place at higher levels in the bureaucracy, matters of
scheduling will be handled at the school level, budgetary
allocation at the school district level, teachers' qualifications
and remuneration at the state or, as in England and France,
at the national levels.

These demographic changes are, to a significant extent,
outside the control of educators. There are changes,
however, which result from educators' conception of their
work. Obviously, coordination in a secondary school is more
complex than in an elementary school because, in the former,
it is thought educationally desirable to specialize by subjects.
This desirability is not seriously questioned by most educators
even though, through team-teaching for example, educators
try to circumvent the more obvious disadvantages of such a
division of labor. The definition of an "educated person" or a
"trained" person also affects the complexity of schools. If an
educated person is thought to require a certain amount of
mathematics in addition to French, physics, etc. then these
activities have to be scheduled through time, sequences have
to be developed, curricula devised, books purchased, equipment ordered, teachers hired, etc. Thus, the socialization
process to a significant degree determines the specialization
or differentiation which will take place in schools and, as I
already argued, such differentiation is very likely to increase
centralization.

Another way of increasing centralization is to focus on
the impact educational organizations have upon their environment. The proportion of GNP devoted to education has increased in virtually all industrialized countries over the last
ten years. In many countries, education represents one of
the largest single expenditures. These increased expenditures
result from increased numbers of students and changing educational needs. However, education must compete with other
societal needs: health, defense, etc. At that time, a greater
scrutiny may take place. Legislators start questioning educational assumptions. The environment becomes less predictable,
no one knowing from year to year whether the budget will be
approved. Under such circumstances, educational organizations
are likely to centralize not only to realize some savings in
terms of administrative ratios, but also in order to control
their operations more closely to show the outsiders that
great care is being used. Evidence shows that an uncertain

environment usually leads to greater centralization and this increased centralization is taking place in a wide variety of educational organizations at the present time: in American universities, in American state departments of education (Milstein and Jennings, 1973) and probably in Europe as well (Benveniste, 1977).

Yet another source of increased centralization is related to socialization. There is not only the curriculum content but the redefinition of the student as a result of research in educational psychology. If the dominant educational assumption claims that only a certain number of children are capable of being educated, then a model curriculum can be developed and little differentiation will take place. If, in addition, the cohort is small and the population socially homogeneous, then differentiation is virtually nonexistent. Thus, in the early part of the twentieth century, the German Gymnasium or the French Lycee were small, socially homogeneous, and had little differentiation; and the whole bureaucratic structure administering secondary education was very simple.

With increased numbers differentiation took place. The limited number of curricula could no longer meet the needs of the expanded population. In addition, this "functional" process of differentiation was reinforced by changing pedagogical assumptions. The learner was seen as a complex individual with special needs. Thus, tne training of teachers has become longer and more complex; and numerous specialists have been hired. Sometimes, legal provisions require that specialists be hired for slow learners, hearing-impaired students, etc. If organizations are shaped by the raw material they are designed to process (Thompson, 1967), a changing definition of that material, in this instance a changing definition of how one learns, would lead to increased complexity of the task or increased specialization. In hospitals "professionalization is directly related to the complexity of the task structure, even when size is controlled" (Heydebrand, 1973:350). This statement probably applies to educational bureaucracies also. The point here is that increased differentiation took place as a result of political and demographic changes over which educators had little or no control. This process has been reinforced by educators as well, i.e., important organizational members have used their beliefs to create or, in this instance, to reinforce, a structure. Changing definitions of what needed to be learned and how one learns led to increases in the size and profes- sionalization of the teaching staff. This increased specializa- tion could lead to increased centralization. These changing definitions required increased financial resources and such demands led to a less stable environment. Unstable environ- ments usually lead to increased centralization as well.

There have been far more forces making for increased centralization in educational bureaucracies than other kinds of forces. This is perhaps what had led many educational critics to view educational bureaucracies as unresponsive, unbending, and interested in certification as opposed to socialization (Meyer, 1977).

Other factors could be mentioned. In the United States, the intervention of the courts and of the federal government in an area which, traditionally has been in the hands of communities certainly has increased centralization. In universities, for example, affirmative-action programs, mandated by law, have tended to remove some of the traditional independence academic departments had in recruiting staff members.

While the intervention of the legal system is perhaps less prevalent in Europe than in the United States, a number of developments have affected centralization there also. In Britain, for example, local education agencies have had, at various times, to submit their plans to the Department of Education and Sciences in London. While not strictly centralizing in nature or intention, the central department nevertheless has increased its power in many areas. In France the monitoring of the labor market is becoming an important matter in educational circles. Quite obviously, such monitoring cannot be done by local communities or by schools. Insofar as the information thus gathered is used to shape certain aspects of educational decisions, then that monitoring can also be considered to be centralizing. These are only illustrations of the factors which reinforce those of size, differentiation and ideology.

EDUCATIONAL BUREAUCRACIES AS LOOSELY
COUPLED SYSTEMS

The picture so far emphasizes organizational structure in a rather mechanical way, i.e., that increased size led to increased centralization, that changes in educational philosophy led to increased differentiation which, in turn, led to increased centralization of decision making. The picture emphasized the connections between the parts of the organization.

It is possible, however, to view organizations, especially educational organizations, as loosely coupled, i.e., as social systems in which the parts are connected but in which they retain their own identity or autonomy (Weick, 1976). It is surely no accident that such a model of educational organizations has been developed in the United States where school systems are loosely coupled and where virtually no formal connections exist at the national level. While it would be easy to describe the French system of education as as structure, it is easy to describe the American system, both at the state and national levels, as loosely coupled. Thus, loose coupling does not apply to schools nor, often, to school districts. The concept applies to the state and national systems.

Five distinct advantages are outlined by Weick as relevant to educational organizations (Weick, 1976:6-8). The first is that "loosely coupled systems . . . 'know' their environments better than is true for more tightly coupled systems."(p. 6).

The concept of local control of schools is an old one in the United States and in England. While, in the United States, the legal authority for education is vested in the state, most states (with the exception of Hawaii) have delegated that responsibility to local authorities. Over the years, states have increased their role, particularly in matters of finance and teacher certification. Nevertheless, the American assumption is that communities constitute the unit most capable of running the schools. While the state may mandate that districts' boundaries be redrawn, the notion that a particular state might be capable of running all schools within its boundaries is unthinkable in the American context. We will later examine the shortcomings of such a system, but in theory as well as in practice, American schools are locally run and the formal connections between school districts within the same state are virtually nonexistent (Wayland, 1973).

A consequence of knowing the environment well is that localized adaptations are possible. Thus, each school district can change its schedule to suit local conditions, can emphasize certain aspects of the curriculum over others (arts over sports, for example), can hire the kinds of teachers it needs, pay them what it wants, determine its particular bureaucratic arrangement, i.e., one which gives either a large or a small amount of control to school principals, etc.

This advantage implies that many educational solutions can exist within American education: very formal schooling, open classrooms, highly selective schools, nonselective ones, etc. Many administrative solutions can also coexist within American education: centralized school systems, decentralized ones, etc.

Furthermore, if a bad or ineffective policy is selected by one school district it does not affect the others. Thus, if the director of elementary schools recommends that reading be taught in a certain way and if it should turn out that that method is ineffective, only children in that school district need be affected. This would be in sharp contrast to the French situation, for example, where all French children would be affected. This is probably why it is possible, in the United States, to receive sometimes a first-rate scientific education, sometimes an indifferent one, and sometimes hardly any at all.

The greater self-determination of loosely coupled systems may lead to a greater sense of efficacy. There is little doubt that in many American communities the school constitutes the most central institution to which everyone belongs or has belonged. It is a social center, and the emotional attachment to that school is strong. People do tend to feel that the school is theirs, and there is substantial involvement on the part of the community members in school affairs. In many instances, the combination of teaching staff-PTA constitutes a special force which the school board cannot easily manipulate. If surveys were available on the subject, there is little doubt that Americans would rank very high on involvement in school affairs.

"A loosely coupled system should be relatively in-expensive to run because it takes time and money to coordinate people" (Weick, 1976:8). While we have seen earlier that increased size led to relatively lower administrative ratios, nevertheless the argument that little coordination need take place in loosely coupled systems is a persuasive one. A look at the number of administrators employed by state educational organizations as well as by school districts reveals that, indeed, the number of supervisory personnel is small. Thus, it may be that loosely coupled systems are relatively inexpensive.

A loosely coupled system presents a number of very significant disadvantages, however. The first can be readily disposed of since, in practice, it does not constitute a problem in the American case. A loosely coupled system is characterized by numerous solutions to educational problems. Successful solutions, because they are localized, cannot readily spread throughout the entire system. This is not a problem because professional organizations and their publications ensure that successful solutions are diffused throughout the entire educational world.

The fact that loosely coupled systems adapt readily to their environment creates the danger of faddish adaptations. More important, however, is that such systems are characterized by great diversity of resources as well as great diversity of results. Weick notes that "loose coupling is a non-rational system of fund allocation" (p. 8) and this particular shortcoming deserves more detailed attention.

Centralization and standardization, the opposite of loose coupling, are methods which facilitate equality. American higher education is decentralized and so is Swiss education. Such systems are characterized by great disparities between schools and between districts. As one indicator, we can note that the Canton of Zurich pays (1975) beginning secondary school teachers about 20 percent more than the Canton of Freiburg, not counting other allowances. At the end of one's career, the pay differential will have increased to 40 percent.

In the United States, some school districts spend $600 a year per student, and one in Texas is reported as spending $7,000 per year. Differences in educational opportunities exist in all countries, but they tend to be greater in decentralized systems than in centralized ones. In France, a highly centralized system, the independent effect of community on educational attainment is virtually nonexistent, while in the United States, such effect is substantially larger (Garnier and Hout, 1976). Local occupational structures obviously affect educational attainment in every society. Thus, communities that are characterized by high-status occupations will exhibit higher than average educational attainment. Whenever comparisons between communities are made concerning the net contribution of educational resources, occupation structure must be controlled.

The relationship between centralization and resource allocation and equality of educational opportunity has not yet been demonstrated. Still, even when efforts at equalization of resources are made, as in Britain, for example, great regional disparities appear (Byrne and Williamson, 1975). The same is true in Germany (Williamson, 1977). Thus, adaptation, flexibility, and responsiveness may be purchased at the cost of substantial inequality.

Localized adaptation may also foster idiosyncratic standards. If no standardization exists, schools can postulate anything as satisfying graduation requirements. The development of standardized testing constitutes a response to this problem in the United States, but many graduates are led to believe that they have received a certain kind of education when, in reality, their achievement is low. In the United States, this situation prevails both at the secondary and university levels.

Localized adaptation may also threaten the intellectual validity of what is being taught. Scientific theories concerning evolution are sometimes challenged because they offend particular religious beliefs. Under such circumstances, the system knows its environment and responds. The response, however, is unlikely to serve the best interests of the students.

By definition, a loosely coupled system is not coordinated. Thus, parts of the system may respond to the immediate environment but may fail to respond to broader or more distant aspects of it. A community may be unaware of changing requirements of the labor force and therefore may fail to adapt its curriculum. Specialized programs can be duplicated or needs may be too small to warrant the development of special programs. It is interesting to note that courts have had to intervene in order to mandate changes which were not desired by local communities; provisions for handicapped children being among them. State educational

agencies are also playing a greater role in making resources
and research findings available. This development often
protects local officials who want such programs but who are
unable to convince the community that they are worth the cost
(Milstein and Jennings, 1973). There is also the possibility
that large districts are better equipped than small ones to
compete for resources such as research grants, experimental
funding from foundations, and the like. Thus, the disparity
between small and large units may be growing. Further, it is
reasonable to assume, and British research shows this to be
the case, that large districts attract more able administrators
than small ones, once again increasing the disparity between
small and large units.

IMPLICATIONS

The structural model of educational administration emphasizes
rationality, hierarchical coordination, and efficiency. The
loosely coupled model emphasizes change, adaptability, local
control. This model also implies that coordination will not be
hierarchical, but rather lateral, when and if it takes place at
all.
     The structural model is comparable with democracy
because bureaucracy is an instrument in the hands of policy
makers. Byrne and Williamson have shown that the party
which controlled the local council in Britain made a difference
as far as educational opportunities were concerned. Chief
education officers can be removed or their life made unpleasant
if they should decide to go against the wishes of the political
leaders (Byrne and Williamson, 1975). Jennings (1977) has
also shown how the educational bureaucracy responded to
political demands. It is reasonable to asuume that it is easier
to control a large but highly structured bureaucracy than one
whose linkages are unknown or nonexistent. Cases where
bureaucracies failed to respond to the demands of a new
administration are probably more rare than is usually assumed.
     The great disadvantage of bureaucratic structures is the
hypothesized rigidity, which implies an inability to change as
well as an inability to respond to local conditions. Such an
assertion is based on a misreading of the literature on
organizational change.
     Early research on organizational change did indeed
indicate that centralization and change were negatively
associated (Hage and Aiken, 1968). More recent evidence,
however, shows that when the organizational elite favors
change, the organization does respond (Hage and Dewar,
1973). Impressionistic evidence indicates that the French
and Swedish educational systems, both highly centralized, have

changed their structure; many of their educational practices have adapted to new situations to an extent not significantly different from the adaptation characteristic of British or American education.

Research on decentralization indicates that many of its hypothesized benefits in fact never materialize (Miller, 1978); school achievement does not increase, and community participation remains at its usual low level.

Does this mean that centralization of control is the answer? Certainly not. Such a solution confuses the issue. The problem with decentralization in the United States is that it takes place without the realization that no matter where control is located, coordination is still required. American education has, so far, failed to establish clear methods of coordination, and thus it may have enjoyed neither the benefits of centralization nor all the benefits of decentralization. Methods of coordination are very informal in American education and, given the uncertain nature of the environment, that informal mechanism may now be inadequate.

It remains the case, however, that "the pluralistic structure of modern organizations presupposes a certain autonomy of subunits" (Heydebrand, 1973:329). That autonomy is probably desirable in education, but coordination is also desirable.

Hierarchical coordination (the traditional bureaucratic solution) is practical under certain circumstances. Such hierarchical coordination is probably desirable in matters of resource allocation. In matters of curriculum, however, the loose structuring prevalent in American education probably offers many substantial benefits. Thus, it would seem that modern educational bureaucracies will have to adopt both types of models within their structures, depending on the particular issue involved. Such a combination of structures is possible only if commitment to the structural model decreases. Education without coordination is problematic. Strictly hierarchical solutions to the problems of coordination are likely to be problematic as well, not only because societies will continue to change, but also because educational research will continue to alter what we know about what needs to be learned and how one learns.

Educational systems in different countries coordinate their activities at different levels. In the American case, coordination rarely takes place, at least in the formal sense. What are the consequences? Low administrative ratios, great inequality, uncertain environment, and therefore prospects for increased centralization in a system ill-designed to accommodate it.

The German case presents a number of interesting possibilities. First, formal coordination takes place hierarchically at the state level. Second, coordination takes

place between the states through the operation of the Kultus
Minister Konferenz (KMK), the Standing Conference of
Ministers of Education. Little research has been done on that
body, which has a secretariat in Bonn, and it would be
worthwhile to determine the consequences of such a body for
the entire system. Within states, there should be fewer
differences between communities in Germany than in the United
States; and differences between states should be somewhat
smaller in Germany than in the United States, if the KMK in
fact operates as an equalizer. Differences can be taken to
mean differences in resources, in educational attainment, or in
any other relevant aspect of education.

For an example of coupling at the national level, one
would turn to the French case. If centralization operates as
an equalizer, France should exhibit the smallest differences
between regions and schools of any system. While it would be
interesting to determine the costs of these different systems,
the problems of measurement are likely to be sufficiently
significant to make such an examination extremely difficult.

A number of dependent variables can be included in this
research model: equality of opportunities, level of attainment,
change, teachers' qualifications, etc.

Given the enormous resources swallowed by education, we
should know more about its administration than is presently
the case. Given that education tends to exhibit great
similarities within national boundaries, only a comparative
design seems possible. Germany has developed an elaborate
system of coordination which is unique and which may be
applicable to the American situation. Learning about its
operation will be useful both to German and American
educators.

8 Modes of Participation and Policy Impact in American Education*
Robert H. Salisbury

There is a pervasive - in modern social-science parlance, paradigmatic - point of view among Americans about how public policy decisions are made. One sophisticated, abstract level of this perspective is expressed by the Eastonian depiction, which holds that environmental circumstances give rise to popular demands, which in turn, are pressed upon the polity's decision-making system.(1) According to this view, there will be no public-policy result unless demands (not to mention supports, both diffuse and specific) are present to provide the efficient stimulus. Demands may result from any or all of several varieties of activity, such as party functions, elections, interest-group lobbying, contacting of citizens, and so on. But whatever the form, the concept of demands clearly rests on the prior assumption that individual citizens will, to some extent and in some fashion, become <u>active</u>, and that by means of their activity, they will create the demands that are a necessary (though not, except to the extremely naive, a sufficient) condition of public-policy outcomes.

Although David Easton intended his formulation to characterize a highly general process, it reflected a distinctively American approach to the concept of citizen's participation. It is not always so apparent to non-Americans that citizen's demands are the motive force from which all policy springs. And this is because it is especially Americans who are entirely suffused with the mythic, metaphorical heritage of John Locke.(2)

*This paper is based in part on work done with the support of grants from the National Institute of Education (NE-G-3-0166) and from Washington University.

In the Lockean world, government derives its just powers from the consent of the governed. Beyond that, however, with the single exception of the conduct of foreign policy,(3) the exercise of those powers is also to be shaped and constrained by the governed. Leaving aside the question of how consent and constraint are effectively to be exercised, there is no doubt that popular judgments are, in the Lockean view, to dominate and give substance to public policy. And there can be little doubt, either, that such judgments must require popular activity to make them explicit and operational. Citizenship itself, both a status and a set of activities, is the primary condition from which all legitimate political action follows. The state, in short, is a derivative of participation.

It is clear that in much of the democratic world such is not the case. Citizenship, in the view of many, is conferred by the state and is dependent upon its wishes.(4) When this view prevails, the place of citizen's participation is theoretically much less central and, indeed, may often be of questionable significance to policy.(5) In the United States, the significance assigned, whether by formula or otherwise, to citizen's participation is absolutely crucial. This tendency has resulted in the creation of many institutional devices and mechanisms whereby citizens do, in fact, take a direct hand in shaping public decisions. Furthermore, rhetorical appeals to the symbols of citizen's participation carry special persuasive power, especially in efforts at "reform." However, much of the participatory activity that takes place may, in fact, be of little policy relevance and may even be a kind of sham. Because participation is so central to the American creed, it is quite likely that many participating citizens are acting out of a kind of patriotic reflex, faithfully doing a duty, the point of which they hardly remember.

This general view has special application to public education in the United States. The school, more than any other institution in American public policy, has depended upon the direct involvement of citizens for its direction and, indeed, its existence. When in 1647 the Massachusetts Bay Colony first mandated the provision of education at public expense, the doctrine of state responsibility for education was articulated.(6) Ever since, the state or its subdivisions, such as the city, county, or school district, has been expected to provide basic education, though at what minimum level has been a matter of continuous dispute.

In fact, however, the provision of schools was left almost entirely to the local community and therefore to the concerned citizens. Whether there would be a school or not, in those early days, depended almost entirely on whether concerned individual citizens mobilized enough support, financial and otherwise, to provide one. Often this effort generated what was virtually a private academy. In the Southern states, the provision of schools was frequently worked out through the Anglican/Episcopalian parish. Indeed, there was little difference in the early days of American education between the levels and types of support by citizens involved in sustaining public schools and those involved in maintaining private schools.(7)

Public education, to be sure, had its base in the legally compulsory taxes extracted from all citizens whether or not they had school-age children. And as the scale and heterogeneity of American communities increased, this connection assumed increasing importance. Yet it should not be forgotten that throughout the nineteenth century in many rural and small-town communities there were few citizens who lacked school-age children. These were young communities with young families that considered the creation of the basic educational machinery their fledgling enterprises, a task of major importance. Legal state control, as opposed to local control, meant almost nothing until the last one hundred years or so. Significant state financial support came even later. American schools had their fundamental basis in the voluntary efforts of the citizens of each particular community. This tradition is not lightly surrendered.

In modern times the tradition has been expressed through several different modes of citizen's participation. First, there is the formal dependence of schools in many states on voter approval of the tax rate that provides financial support of the local community. Although there is much variation from one state to another in the frequency of direct referendum-type elections governing school-policy matters, only two of the fifty states make no use of them at all.(8) Beyond this formal support there is a substantial degree of dependence by many schools on informal support in the form of supplementary fund raising and direct auxiliary services. It is extremely difficult to estimate how much of this kind of participation there is or how much it contributes to educational programs, but it is not trivial.

Like most governments in the United States, schools are governed by citizens, whether elected or appointed, who participate without significant reimbursement. This reliance on activism by citizens for policy guidance is one of the most cherished prerogatives in the American political tradition, and it is linked to some deeply rooted values - the superior virtue of local control, for example, and the importance of maintaining lay rather than professional control over school affairs.

A further function of participation by citizens is implicit in the principle of governance by citizens. It is mainly through the activity of citizens that community norms and expectations regarding educational policy are articulated and pressed upon school officials. School professionals have often lamented such activity, calling it pressure, contending that it

may result in distortions of sound educational practice.
Conversely, it has been through demands of citizens that many
recent changes in educational priorities have been brought
about, the changes with regard to racial integration in
American cities being the most dramatic. Whatever the value
different groups may ascribe to demands, the involvement of
citizens remains a basic mechanism, though not the only one,
through the use of which the substance of educational
programs is determined. Furthermore, it should not be
overlooked that participatory pressure is exerted in many
directions. Private citizens have both sought to block the
teaching of sex education and sought to bring about
educational equality for racial minorities. Citizens both urge
and oppose school busing for racial integration. There has
seldom been agreement for the direction of policy resulting
from the involvement of citizens in education, and there has
seldom been much vitality in American education without the
active participation of large numbers of ordinary citizens.

TYPES OF PARTICIPATION

Some of the most important, recent literature dealing with
participation has been concerned with establishing the
categories or types within which participatory behavior falls.
The work of Verba and Nie is the best of such efforts. It is
useful to consider what they have done both in contrast to
what had come before and in its relation to school-centered
participation.(9) Until the Verba-Nie work, the prevailing
view was that political participation was unidimensional.(10)
It ranged, for any set of actors, from much to little, with all
political thought to lie along this quantitative dimension. What
Verba and Nie showed was the several distinct dimensions
involved. Just because a person was active in electoral
politics, for example, did not mean that he or she was active
in community affairs, and vice versa. Verba and Nie
concluded that there were four distinct types of activity:
voting, electoral campaigning, communal involvement, and
personal contact with officials; they also concluded that these
corresponded to six types of participants: those specializing in
one or another of the four activity sets, those who were
altogether inactive, and those who were active in all areas.
To at least some extent, both the unidimensional line of
research and the Verba and Nie revision have displayed a
generic tendency of social science to obtain only those
empirical results predicted by the forms of the questions
asked. Verba and Nie, for example, excluded protest
demonstrations and other "irregular" modes of participation.
Consequently, they found no protester type in their data.

Similarly, the older research had asked only about election-centered behavior(11) and therefore found no evidence of communalist participation. Nevertheless, Verba and Nie have not been modest in asserting the general applicability of their typology. And since they have secured essentially similar responses to the same set of questions in the several other nations they have surveyed,(12) they have felt quite comfortable in this conviction.

A case can be made that the Verba-Nie line of analysis in fact places its participation types within one of two more or less distinct institutional boundaries, those delineating partisan elections on the one hand, and those marking community affairs on the other. Insofar as this may be true, it might well be that an investigation of other institutional settings would turn up sets of people who were quite active in one or more of those settings although not active in the ones Verba and Nie asked about. It is certainly as reasonable to expect to find active school specialists or church specialists as it is to find election campaign specialists. This point is of particular importance if we wish to understand participation related to schools and to attempt to draw inferences from the Verba-Nie findings.

A second consideration to be borne in mind regarding the Verba-Nie formulation is that it presupposes that participation is purposive. Participation, Verba and Nie contend, consists of those acts intended to affect the policy decisions of government. Leaving aside whether this definition does not assume far too much rationalism on the part of ordinary voters, it plainly excludes from view much activity that we might well want to examine in a study of participation. When an individual joins an organization such as the neighborhood school PTA, for example, it is seldom clear that he or she does so in order to affect school policy. Yet, having joined, people may find themselves well situated to mobilize influence if, someday, they wish to exert it. The joining of groups and the exertion of policy influence through those groups are conceptually and empirically distinct.(13) Often, one type of behavior may be converted into the other when circumstances warrant, and the connections and relationships between purposive and nonpurposive behavior are very much worth investigating. They must not be excluded by too narrow a definition.

CITIZEN-PARTICIPANTS IN EDUCATION

Research has recently been completed involving rather lengthy interviews with some 507 school activists in six suburban school districts in the St. Louis, Missouri, metropolitan area.

Respondents were chosen from among those who displayed at least a minimum level of participatory activity, such as attending school organization meetings.

There are many distinct forms that citizen participation in school affairs may take, and the most common is membership in a school-related group. In 1974 an NORC survey reported that 17.5 percent of American adults belonged to some school organization. This figure is astonishingly high; it represents roughly twenty-two million people. But it only begins to indicate the size of the number of Americans who take some kind of active part in school affairs. It is not wholly clear what is included in this broad set of activities, but there has been a formidable number of people who march in the streets, contribute time or money to school election campaigns, participate in ad hoc or informal groups, or even go to court to seek redress. Many of these people are purposive participants; they do indeed seek to affect educational policy through their activity. Their desires may often be disappointed, and they may or may not persist in their endeavors. Their efforts embody the traditions of citizen effort, for their whole socialization has led them, often with exaggerated expectations, to believe that the mere fact that they try will be sufficient to effect the desired result.

Purposive participation indicates that there is some degree of unhappiness with the way things are and that the citizen wants to change things either for his or her own children or, in more abstract terms, for the general welfare. This observation leads us to ask about the processes by which citizens are induced to play an active role. Virtually without exception, school activists are brought into initial involvement at the time of the entrance of their oldest children into school. Regardless of whether or not the involvement blossoms into a purposive crusade, it begins with the children's entrance into school. Thereafter, some fractions of the parents become dissatisfied and seek to change or to prevent change in their children's schooling. Another fraction, however, which is often larger than the other, seeks only to provide support for the schools as they are.

The amount of supportive participation may vary from much to little. There can be quite a frenetic pace, as class mothers drive car pools on field trips, sew school-play costumes, bake cookies, and otherwise display their parental devotion. In the same fashion, purposive participation may also range from less to more. Indeed, unless one probes the specific motivations, it may be difficult to distinguish between the lethargic purposive activist and the modestly enthusiastic supporter of the schools. It is at the high levels of activity that the difference between the kinds of activity is marked. The supportive enthusiast is uncritical and spends much time on his or her activities. The purposive activist has policy goals that PTA or committee or electoral work is to accomplish.

What factors account for the different types and amounts of school-related participation? The St. Louis data provide a somewhat more complete set of answers than most other studies. First, there is almost no support for the argument that elements in the family background and/or socialization leads people toward greater or lesser amounts of school participation. No really significant relationships were found between parental interest or involvement in school affairs and corresponding participation levels. Second, there was a substantial class effect. Less affluent and/or less well-educated people participated less intensely, ceteris paribus, than those higher on the socioeconomic status ladder. St. Louis-area school participants generally were significantly higher in socioeconomic rank than the socioeconomic status median for their communities, a finding highly similar to ones in nearly every national study of participation.

One conclusion that follows from this material is that those communities whose members are of higher than average social rank have larger amounts of citizen activism. Conversely, communities of lower socioeconomic status standing, such as most cities in the United States, have considerably less citizen involvement.

School-centered participation has historically been the special province of women. In most areas of public life women participate less than men, a fact that has been taken to support the allegation that women occupy a prejudicially subordinate place in American society. The schools are an exception, or at least they appear to be, for two-thirds of the school activists in St. Louis and elsewhere are women. On closer inspection, however, it turns out that the motivation of women to participate is routine and almost reflexive and that their participation is disproportionately supportive. Women are brought into school-related activity by their role as parents, but they are not provoked in these roles to seek policy changes. Nor, for the most part, do they seek to rise through some hierarchy of participatory effort to positions of prominence and putative influence. At the upper levels of school participation, men occupy a much larger share of the important positions. So even in an arena that traditionally has been identified as "women's work," men dominate the positions of real importance.(14)

This observation raises a question of fundamental importance. What significance is to be attributed to the various forms and levels of participation? Are the lower levels of intensity to be viewed as mere window dressing? Or, for that matter, do the upper levels, such as school board or citizens committee membership, really carry effective power? It is certainly possible that although these positions are dominated by men, this domination reflects not the impor-tance of the offices, but rather a social tradition that to a disproportionate degree places men in high office or induces men to seek high office.

There are at least three quite distinct kinds of impact of community characteristics on the patterns of school-related participation by citizens. First, there is the effect of socio-economic status, which has already been noted. It is quite clear that communities with a high-median social rank have more participation than less affluent ones. Size of the community may be a factor that reinforces this tendency, but neither the St. Louis data nor national surveys permit a close analysis. It is reasonable, however, to suppose that the larger the community, the less participatory its citizens will be inclined to be, both because of the presumably greater atomization and alienation of big city life and because the authorities are more remote and insulated from effective pressure. It is not simply the socioeconomic status distribution in a community that is of relevance, of course. Demographic trends (rising or falling enrollment, for example), social heterogeneity (many patterns of variations may still result in a common mean), and subtle subcultural attitudes regarding education all have their effects.

The structure of the community may be of significance. School district boundaries do not always coincide with the boundaries of municipalities. In the St. Louis study, one school district was composed of twenty-three separate municipalities, while another included considerable farm country surrounding a town. Such structures reduce participation in at least two ways. Citizens do not know where to turn with complaints since the authorities to which they must appeal have differing structures and are far away. In addition, there are fewer opportunities for interaction among the members of the school district, since so much social business takes place within the smaller, municipal divisions. Civic knowledge and social interaction both contribute to the ease and likelihood of further participation.

Complexity and confusion in the structure of public authority, the hallmarks of American governmental design, inhibit citizen participation. And, it may be noted, legislative mandates for the increase of participation through the creation of ad hoc mechanisms for local participation in schools, poverty programs, or community development may in the long run exacerbate this inhibition.

An additional structural factor is related to the methods of selection of the school board and approval of the school tax. If these processes are closely tied to the broader political processes of the community - if, for example, the mayor appoints the school board - then school-related participation will be part of a larger pattern of community involvement. If, however, as is more common, school governance is structurally separated, school participation is much more likely to be the province of school specialists.

PERGAMON PRESS, INC.

INTERNATIONAL PUBLISHERS OF SCIENTIFIC BOOKS & JOURNALS
NEW YORK * OXFORD * TORONTO * SYDNEY

We are pleased to send to you enclosed
a complimentary copy of the following book for review:

COMPARATIVE PUBLIC POLICY & CITIZENS
   PARTICIPATION
Foster
ISBN 0 08 024624 9 hardcover $27.50
Published February 1980

(1) 024624 9 to be sent by 31 March 80
50/R

Published/Distributed by
   ☒ Pergamon Press, Inc. ☐ Pergamon of Canada, Ltd.
   ☐ British Book Centre/Div. Pergamon Press, Inc.
Please send two copies of your review to:

Promotion Manager
Pergamon Press, Inc.
Maxwell House, Fairview Park
Elmsford, New York 10523   Printed in U.S.A.

A third element of the effect of the characteristics of the community is to be found in the context of issues. Each community or school district has a history that. is in some respects unique. Some communities, for explicable but subtly combined historical reasons, place an especially strong emphasis on the quality of their schools. They attract residents partly because of that emphasis who, in turn, take a comparatively more active role in order to preserve the reputation of the community and the corresponding property values. In some communities, the schools become the battleground between the old and the new generations of settlers, between adherents to differing social philosophies, or, most visibly and dramatically, between different racial or ethnic groups. Such conflicts not only have historical consequences, but may also have profound social and economic effects. There were, for example, the melodramas associated with racial change in American and British schools.

We should not conclude that each school district is so distinctive that no general statements about who governs and why can be made. There are, however, differences among any group of school districts in the amount and kind of participation there is. For example, in two of the St. Louis districts the active participants were quite similar in socioeconomic background and situation. One district, however, enjoyed a considerably larger tax base, while the other contained a significant minority of black students. The latter district faced the necessity of reorganizing if it was to bring about racial balance. In the other district there really were no problems, crises, or even dissatisfactions. Not surprisingly, the consequence was that in the problem-free district participation was substantial and uncritically supportive (because of the high socioeconomic status level) while in the other case, where participants were drawn from very similar school strata, their involvement was highly purposive, intended to change school policy.

Surely, this similarity is not a random result. The socioeconomic status factor of one community prescribed the level of participation there, while the community context prescribed the substantive focus of the other. Although the particular combinations are unique, the variables are generic. There are two points to be remembered. First, there are not enough carefully examined cases to make entirely clear what are the central variables. Class composition and the legacy of community conflict are certainly important almost everywhere in their influence on school-related participation. But there may also be other relevant factors. The St. Louis study identified some of these, such as structural integration of the community and rates of community growth and change. Second, it seems very likely that in the United States the level and charac- ter of citizen participation in the schools is vitally shaped by circumstances in the local community rather than those in the state, region, or nation. Contextual factors operating through interpersonal networks on the community level are of crucial importance, and in this respect the American case may be substantially different from European counterparts.

One mode of citizens' participation in American school affairs is membership on citizens' committees, usually acquired through appointment by the mayor, school board, or school superintendent. These committees may be designed to provide an official examination of a school problem, general citizen's counsel on school affairs, or perhaps legitimation of school policies. Unlike the school boards, these committees do not set policy. Compared to the ordinary forms of participation, membership on such committees involves much heavier commitments of time and attention. Sometimes citizen committee members have been co-opted, of course. They are allowed to participate so they can be seduced into giving support which otherwise might not have been given to the educational status quo. Some fraction of this group, however, learns to be critical, developing in the course of their committee service a more exacting standard of what public education ought to be. The St. Louis data indicate that although citizen committee members display considerable diversity, they tend, in the aggregate, to be somewhat more critical of the schools and to be more affected by their participatory experience than those who engage in the more routine participatory activities of parent organizations.

Still more substantial impact from school participation is reported by those who run for and serve on school boards. They are, of course, a very small fraction of the total population, but there are nearly 16,000 local school boards and the total number of people serving at any one time is in the vicinity of 90,000.(15) Board members, though unpaid, devote large amounts of time to the job. In very few cases do those who serve on school boards seem to have any sort of further ambitions. Their motivations, at least those that are conscious and explicit, are feelings of citizen's duty, the desire to serve children and the community, and a degree of intellectual interest in the affairs of the public schools. What is perhaps most instructive is that board members are more likely than other types of participants to report that their opinion of the schools has changed for the better. Familiarity seems on the whole to breed approval rather than contempt, and this raises a question of great importance. Does more active participation enhance attitudes that are supportive of the existing situation, or can activism be an efficient mechanism for bringing about change? The St. Louis data suggest that for the most part participation leads to support, regardless of how critical participants may be of specific details, and that, therefore, the more activism there is ceteris paribus, the stronger the existing institutions and practices will be.

The discussion thus far has perhaps implied that school-related participation takes place only at the local level and only with normal structural arrangements. This is usually true, but it is not exclusively so. One arena of participation, for example, has been the White House Conference on Education, held at national and state levels from time to time since the 1950s, which is designed to mold and rally elite opinion in support of public education.(16) Sometimes curriculum reform has also been included in the programs. This method of elite mobilization, usually conducted by executive branch officials, is also common in such policy areas as foreign affairs.(17) There is little evidence that much "trickle down" of influence occurs. Mass opinion is not much affected. But within the elite itself there may well be a legacy of enthusiasm, even of zealotry, that motivates a small number of highly active influential people. Their activity may well be enough to alter some aspects of public policy.

If insistent individuals can sometimes affect school policy, so can protesting groups who express their concerns outside the normal channels, taking to the streets or the picket lines.(18) Few policy sectors have been more obviously or profoundly affected by protest activity of citizens than has education. The protests have been particularly fierce over racial integration. At another, very different level, United States school activists practically invented the strategy, later emulated by environmentalists and others, of using the courts to secure their policy desires.(19) Still another mode of citizen involvement is working through organized interest groups such as the National Education Association, the Council on Basic Education, or the Citizens for Educational Freedom. Such groups often lobby at the national level, and they are the chief means by which activism of citizens is brought to bear on state and national educational policy.(20)

One must keep in mind that citizen participation is, among other things, a strategy for pursuing policy objectives. Eliciting participation is easier when one's policy cause draws broad, or at least intensely felt, popular support. The arenas of participation are decided by which participatory resources of the group are most readily mobilized, regardless of whether or not they are the most efficient. Thus, it may be appealing to mobilize a crowd even though the decision on the issue at hand is to be made in court.(21) Although American civic tradition does not fully accept the fact there can be no assumption that simply because citizens take some action - whether it be a protest march, a tax vote, a lobbying effort, a petition to the school board, a mass meeting, or an election campaign - they will win. Active citizens can and do lose, just as do those who remain inactive.(22)

IMPACT OF PARTICIPATION ON THE PARTICIPANT

The primary objective of the St. Louis study was to
investigate the impact that participation has on the participant.
It sought to determine whether such scholars as Aristotle and
John Stuart Mill were correct in asserting that active citizens
are changed by their activity. The impact of activity on
people can take several forms. It may simply be the
acquisition of new information or it may be a change of one's
attitudes and opinions. It might lead to new patterns of social
interaction or to expanded participation in other organizational
settings. The impact might also entail, as Mill expected, some
transformation of the self, enhanced personal capacities, or a
growth in self-confidence. The problems of measuring this
impact are formidable. The impact is both subtle and complex
in its manifestations. Much of the impact expected to result
from participation may appear only several years later, and
without good data the ability to identify the effects of impact
and sort out causal connections is limited. Nevertheless,
respondents were asked a variety of different types of
questions bearing on the matter of the impact of activity, and
the findings may be of interest.
     Participation, even at a relatively modest level, does
result in opinion change. Different formulations of the
question produced different proportions of affirmative
responses, but never less than one-third answered positively.
More interesting was the direction of this change in opinion.
Those who reported changing their opinions as a result of
their involvement were more critical of the schools than those
who remained unaffected by their experience. Thus, the
earlier comment about the continued supportiveness of highly
involved citizens requires some modification. Substantial
proportions of school participants reported that they had
gained information and grown personally through participation.
The more active the respondents were, the more likely they
were to stress that they had grown personally, which suggests
that Mill was indeed correct.
     There are long-term effects of school participation on
involvement in other organizations, but assessment of them is a
bit complicated. The data show clearly that a sizable fraction
of school activists expect to move into other civic activity once
their children are out of school and the school arena no longer
interests them. The close connection between the age
structure of the family and both entry into and exit from
school participation gives these citizens who have children in
school a distinctive character. The more active they are in
school affairs, the more likely they are to move subsequently
into other community arenas. Thus, the schools become
something of a springboard for civic participation in general.

Many of the people who follow this course, however, are individuals who, by reason of their social class and particular histories and inclinations, would have been likely to become active in the community even if they had been childless and hence not concerned about schools. Only a small fraction can be said to have moved into broader civic participation because of their experience in school affairs. Yet even this handful, accumulating over time, may have a significant renewing effect on a community's activist elite. In any event, more careful consideration must be given to the overlapping patterns of participation in different arenas of public life and, in particular, to how these change through time.(23)

There is another relationship that may very well represent an effect of participation and that reveals an important dimension of the attitudes of school activists about the political world. In the St. Louis study, there were a series of questions, adapted from other surveys, that sought to measure what is generally referred to as "trust in government." These questions were asked separately about each of five levels of government: national, state, county, city, and school district. There are some complexities in the data, but the main result is undeniable. The school districts are the most trusted level of government. Beyond this, however,the smaller and less removed the governmental unit was, the more trusted it was. In the immediate post-Watergate period it is not surprising that the national government was trusted the least. It is more significant that the schools, and after them local government, were ranked most trustworthy. Moreover, the respondents felt the trustworthiness of these local levels of government to be very high. It seems clear that the amount and intensity of participation is closely linked to approval of the level of government at which one is to participate.

In these days of precipitate decline of popular trust, it may be especially important to take this finding seriously. If participants are trusting and confident and cynics remain on the sidelines, then the motivations for involvement transcend the pursuit of self-interest or the enhancement of self-confidence and individual capability. In this light, participation can be seen as an important mechanism by which to strengthen popular belief in, and support for, the essential governing processes of the society.

FRAMEWORK FOR PARTICIPATION

The research on school participation can be placed in a much broader context and participation can be related to some factors not previously mentioned. These relationships can be illustrated in a two-dimensional matrix (figure 8.1). Along one axis are progressive degrees of institutionalization. This variable measures the extent to which participatory activity is shaped and constrained by the rules of a formally constituted arena or regulated according to a bureaucratic code of appropriate practice. Participation in a court, for instance, is an activity that is highly regulated, while joining in a street demonstration is one that is not.

On the other axis, the levels of motivation of participants are arranged according to the extent to which they reflect autonomous personal values as opposed to participatory pressures from a group or from a legally imposed mandate.

In the lower left-hand corner is the ideal condition in which citizens join together freely and of their own volition, without the constraint of rules or even specialized roles, to cooperate and solve common problems. In the opposite corner is the condition which results in the antithesis of spontaneous citizen action; in this condition, people act only because they are required to, and they are heavily restricted in what they may do and how they may do it by an entrenched bureaucracy. Observers of citizens' involvement in West German school affairs seemed to believe that it was an example of participation under this highly constrained condition.

Parental participation in the United States, on the other hand, would rank quite high on the scale of autonomy of motivation. Most parents begin participating, as we have seen, because their children have started school, and they feel an obligation to assist their children's education by joining the PTA and supporting the school program. Cultural backgrounds and socialization processes no doubt have operated to bring a disproportionate share of the well-educated middle class into participation, but there the relevant factors are individual attitudes rather than group pressure or government edicts. American school participation does occur within an institutional framework composed of the schools themselves and the mechanisms discussed earlier, such as the PTA and organizations involved in a school-tax campaign. But these organizations tend to be quite loose and are often poorly differentiated, and their vigor is likely to ebb and flow with events and personalities. Indeed, in many areas of American political life the institutional arenas are not very sharply delineated. They are shadowy areas at the peripheries that give rise to uncertainty as to just what can be expected. This quality is certainly characteristic of the party system in general and of some parts of the legislative process and the executive branch; it is also typical of state and local levels of government. Hence it is probably reasonable to place the majority of American political activity in the middle sections of the matrix.

MOTIVATIONAL AUTONOMY

	Low	Medium	High
Low (Mandated Pressure)			Bureaucratized and Mandated; Citizens in West German Schools
Medium (Group Pressure)		Interest-Group Lobbying	Corporatist Policy Making
High (Personal Values)	Radical Ideal	U.S. Parental Participation	"Sue 'em"

INSTITUTIONALIZATION

Figure 8.1

The Matrix of Citizen Participation

The only exceptions are the courts. The judicial arena is highly institutionalized; however, the motivations that lead people to enter this arena may be highly personal and individual. The litigiousness of people varies with time and circumstance, but it, too, is a type of participation.

The use of the illustrative scheme has been limited mainly to education-related participation, but it seems that it is not necessary to thus limit its application. The basic variables of institutionalization and motivational autonomy are appropriate to the analysis of almost any political system. Further, variations in the amount as well as the type of participation could be incorporated by adding a third dimension.

What purpose is served by this schema? First, it calls attention to the importance of the relationship between individual motivations and the institutional context in which they are felt. Second, it indicates the importance of identifying and mapping the variety of interests and motives that lead people into political participation. It is truly astonishing that so little attention has been given to determining what purposes are served by citizen's action. The argument presented here insists that different purposes pursued in different institutional arenas will yield quite different patterns of participation.

It is possible that there are theoretical linkages between this kind of formulation of patterns of participation and the somewhat similar schemas developed elsewhere of the pattern of public policy.(24) In both cases it is the interaction between values or interests and institutional structure that is critical.

NOTES

(1)   Perhaps we would have come to some such formulation anyway, but it is David Easton's schema that has defined the world within which political science that is policy-oriented has worked for two decades. A Systems Analysis of Political Life (New York: Wiley, 1965).

(2)   Louis Hartz's explication of this argument remains persuasive. The Liberal Tradition in America (New York: Knopf, 1955), and "Democracy: Image and Reality," in Wm. H. Chambers and Robert H. Salisbury, Democracy in the Mid-Twentieth Century (St. Louis: Washington University Press, 1960).

(3)   See Locke's Second Treatise of Civil Government, Ch. XII.

(4)   See T.H. Marshall, Class, Citizenship and Social Development, (Garden City: Doubleday, 1965).

(5)   Recent discussions of the significance of participation in democratic politics seem to have missed this point. See,

inter alia, Carole Pateman, Participation and Democratic Theory (Cambridge: Cambridge University Press, 1970); Dennis Thompson, The Democratic Citizen (Cambridge: Cambridge University Press, 1970).

(6)   It is hoped that the reader will be able to recognize the distinction made in the use of the term state. Here we are using it in the American context, meaning the major units of the federal system, rather than as a generic term for authoritative government.

(7)   On the history of American education, generally, see R. Freeman Butts and Lawrence A. Cremin, A History of Education in the United States (New York: Henry Holt, 1953).

(8)   See Howard Hamilton and Sylvan Cohen, Policy-Making by Plebiscite: School Referenda (Lexington Books, 1975).

(9)   Participation in America: Political Democracy and Social Equality (New York: Harper and Row, 1972).

(10) See, for example, Lester Milbrath, Political Participation (Rand McNally, 1965). But cf. the revised edition, with Goel, 1977.

(11) The most substantial data sets were generated by the Survey Research Center's biennial polls.

(12) See Verba, Nie, and Kim, The Modes of Democratic Participation: A Cross-National Analysis, Sage, 1971, and by the same authors, Participation and Political Equality (Cambridge: Cambridge University Press, 1978).

(13) The classic statement of this argument is, of course, Mancur Olson, The Logic Of Collective Action (Cambridge, Mass.: Harvard University Press, 1965). See also my "An Exchange Theory of Interest Groups," Midwest Journal of Political Science vol 11, p. 1310 (February, 1969).

(14) We would not wish this conclusion to imply support for a sexist view. In fact, if education and experience are controlled, women appear to hold their own even at higher levels of school participation. But many more of the supportive participants are women.

(15) See Harmon Ziegler and Kent Jennings, Governing American Schools (North Scitnate: Duxbury Press, 1974).

(16) See George Grassmuck, "The White Conference in Education," presented at the 1977 meeting of the Midwest Political Science Association.

(17) See James Rosenau, National Leadership and Foreign Policy: A Case Study in the Mobilization of Public Support (Princeton: Princeton University Press, 1963).

(18) See Michael Lipsky, "Protest as a Political Resource," American Political Science Review vol. (LXII) (December, 1968).

(19) See the magisterial work by Richard Kluger, Simple Justice (New York: Knopf, 1975).

(20)   See the relatively recent discussion of school lobbies in
       Congressional Quarterly,   The Washington Lobby,   2nd
       ed., 1978.

(21)   It is instructive to note the Spring, 1978, demonstra-
       tions articulating the desire of blacks and others to
       obtain a favorable outcome in the historic Bakke case,
       which involved so-called reverse discrimination.

(22)   A profoundly important finding apropos of this point is
       John Mueller's report that American public opinion fol-
       lowed almost exactly the same curve of increasing dis-
       approval during the Vietnam War as it had during the
       Korean War.   In the latter case there were few protests
       or sit-ins, but in both instances opinion changed as a
       logarithmic function of the casualty rate.   See War,
       Presidents and Public Opinion, 1973.

(23)   See my unpublished paper "Overlapping Memberships,
       Organizational Interactions, and Interest Group Theory,"
       presented to the American Political Science Association,
       1976.

(24)   Two papers of mine have explored these relationships as
       they apply to the analysis of public policy: "The Analysis
       of Public Policy: Search for Theory and Roles," in Austin
       Ranney,   ed.,   Political Science and Public Policy   (San
       Francisco: Markham, 1968); and with J.P. Heinz, "A
       Theory of Policy Analysis and Some Preliminary Applica-
       tions," in Ira Sharkansky, ed., Policy Analysis in
       Political Science (San Francisco: Markham, 1970).

9 Teachers and Participation: Experiences with Participation in the Continuing Education of Teachers in West Germany

Raimund Klauser

Participation in the educational system of the Federal Republic of Germany cannot be easily defined. Educational policy there is determined mainly by the respective federal states. In spite of the hierarchic-bureaucratic organization of the educational administration, educational policy is characterized by such complicated substructures of both institutions and areas of authority that it is extremely difficult to find a consistent concept of participation based on a democratic theory.

The same is true of the system of continuing education of teachers, which has too often been neglected in the vehement debate over participation in the educational system. Nevertheless, there have been repeated efforts to define and put into practice a demand for participation in this area.

Given the number of institutions dealing with the continuing education of teachers and the number of courses offered by these institutions, experiments in participation have been relatively rare; only in a few cases have they been planned and realized with consistency. However, there has always been a fundamental problem: the expectations connected with the demand for participation are extremely high but can seldom be fully realized.

Polarity is evident between the demand for participation derived from a democratic theory and corresponding concepts of action and a distinct pragmatism which is supposed to aid practical participation in continuing education.

PROBLEMS OF PARTICIPATION

As experience shows, there is a sharp contrast between a theoretical demand for participation and the practical pos-

117

sibilities of real participation. This problem is by no means restricted to the educational system.

In analyzing policy processes it is important to keep in mind that an individual acting politically bases his perceptions and ideas for solving problems on only those perceptions and ideas for solution that he has had before. This fact leads to the conclusion that the entire issue of participation can be examined only if the aims of participation that have been formulated abstractly are contrasted with the specific experiences, opportunities for action, and interests of the participants. Through such an examination, a way of mediation must be found.

In the continuing education of teachers, particular care should be taken in finding a way for mediation, since this kind of education has to fulfill two important tasks: It is supposed to ensure and increase the teacher's professional qualifications for adequate instruction, and it is to provide additional qualifications that are likely to further the teacher's career.

These goals can be reached only if the teachers' experiences, opportunities for action, and interests are taken into account in determining subject matter and in organizing a project. This requires participation. Also, if teachers and students are to cooperate, it is essential that the teacher be qualified for such cooperation. Thus, methods of participation are themselves a subject in the continuing education of teachers.

If participation is proposed in the continuing education of teachers, and if a first step toward the realization of this proposal is to be establishing mechanisms for participation in decision making, the institution of such mechanisms must be such that the resultant participation is appropriate to the needs of the teachers involved.

This sets high standards for the model of participation on which the continuing education is to be based; it also requires the teachers to be prepared to make use of the opportunity for participation.

But what have been the experiences with participation in the Federal Republic of Germany? What happened when people tried to realize participation beyond institutionalized forms such as voting? What happened when they tried to legitimate political decisions and to improve the quality of political decisions, thereby hoping to realize the democratic norm of individual and collective self-determination by citizens?

In many political fields participation models were conceived once the legal foundations had been laid. These models took into full consideration the interests of the citizens and the possibilities for action - or so the authors of such models maintain. When processes of participation were put into practice, however, there was always a great difference between the theories and their realization. The repeated failures of participation models (especially in those cases that involved contrasting interests of the political administration and the citizens) indicate that in many cases participation has been misunderstood. Attempts at participation failed because the underlying notion of participation and its transformation into a practical model did not accurately comprehend the individual possibilities for perception and action of those citizens who should (and would) participate. A number of examples can be given for this phenomenon in the field of town planning and in the various sectors of educational policy.

German teachers' experiences with participation have been poor. Willingness to participate can be expected of them only if they are offered a practicable theory of participation and a concrete plan for action. The necessity of practicality must be emphasized, especially since at present new laws concerning participation are being prepared or put into practice in several states of the Federal Republic. These laws will help to give teachers a chance for participation. Nevertheless, teachers will continue to demand more opportunities for participation.

A second problem area is closely connected with the problem of the differences between the demand for and the opportunities for participation. The continuing education of teachers has a central function in the innovation of the educational system. Innovations concerning the curriculum must be conveyed to the teacher in such a way that he can act according to them if they are expected to have any effect in the classroom. The teacher must therefore be able to think over the goals and subject matter of these innovations and to identify himself with them and organize his lessons accordingly. Curricular innovations always depend on the agreement of the teachers, for otherwise they are bound to fail.(1) Given that its task is to continually ensure and improve the teachers' qualifications for their profession, continuing education of teachers should take upon itself the responsibility for this process of mediation.

The demand for participation in the process of curricular innovations can indeed be met in reality. As a rule, the teachers' consent to an innovation is given if the continuing-education programs are adequate. But is this kind of participation nothing more than passive assent by the teachers? Under such conditions, the qualification of teachers to participate actively can by no means be achieved.

It has become obvious that the definition of the role of the continuing education of teachers in the process of curricular innovation has been changed. In connection with this change, the demand for participation has been raised. In the educational system of West Germany, curricula are in most cases still developed by a central commission and then introduced into the schools. In some cases, the continuing education of teachers is meant to lead to revisions of the

curricula. The teachers who are to work with the new
curriculum are supposed to participate in such a way that they
develop bases for making such revision during their continuing
education period. The demand for such participation and its
reality, however, are by no means without contradictions.
    In 1973, " Richtlinien fur den Politik - Unterricht" (A
Framework for Political Education), was introduced in schools
in the federal state of North-Rhine-Westphalia. These
guidelines form only a curricular framework the implementation
of which requires special training for the teacher. To spread
this innovation, a special system of dissemination was
conceived, a system that was to function through the
continuing education of teachers. The content of this
curriculum was ambitious. It included the notion of broad
participation based on the right of self-determination. The
teaching of political participation itself was to be an integral
part of the curriculum. Teachers were asked to try out the
curriculum, and to articulate their experiences that would aid
in the making of a possible revision.
    In reality, however, this plan did not provide for
participation. The curriculum was designed by a commission in
which teachers actually working in schools were
underrepresented. As is usual in the West German educational
system, the curriculum was prescribed for all teachers, and so
there was no opportunity for an individual teacher to reject
the curricular innovation. The system of dissemination built
into the central and regional continuing education of teachers
did not work. This was due not only to fundamental
deficiencies in the concept of dissemination itself, but also to
the total lack of opportunities for participation for teachers in
the making of decisions concerning subject matter and
methods. Neither in the continuing education of teachers nor
in individual schools were any foundations for the revision of
the curriculum developed. Furthermore, the school
administration showed no particular interest in making any
revisions.
    The school administration did not even make an effort to
put into practice the maintained demand for participation.
This failure was one of the primary reasons for the failure of
their efforts to introduce a new curricular framework. The
teachers became extremely suspicious of the demand for
participation in the revision of curriculum. The curriculum as
a whole was regarded as politically inconsistent and
implausible, and many teachers "participated" by not using the
curriculum in their lessons.
    This example illustrates that the failure to realize or to
realize sufficiently the demand for participation in the process
of curricular innovation can inhibit the teacher's motivation.
It can even lead to a certain hostility toward participation if
the teacher is not offered any real opportunities for input.
This hostility is difficult to appease.

A third field of problems involves the organization of the continuing education of teachers on the basis of participation. The functioning educational system and the realization of the goals of educational policy in the schools depend on the teachers' readiness to cooperate. In this connection, participation can act as an aid in the establishment of this readiness for cooperation.(2) The question is whether the present continuing education of teachers includes a sufficient number of decision-making and participation-oriented structures to make the teachers want to cooperate.

Apart from a few exceptions, such structures are missing completely. Still, both school administrations and various other institutions concerned with the continuing education of teachers maintain that the individual teacher has extensive opportunities to influence decisions concerning the subject matter and methods of continuing education. In reality, the opposite is true in most cases; the goals and subject matter of the continuing education of teachers are in most cases defined by the school administration or the particular institution without the cooperation of the teachers. Moreover, the aims and subject matter are often far removed from the needs and interests of the teachers. The school administration even decides which teachers are to take courses in continuing education.

In these courses the teacher is offered few opportunities for initiative. Teachers are put under great strain because while intensive participation is demanded of them, all their experiences with it are negative.

IMPROVING TEACHER PARTICIPATION

Teachers are seldom motivated or qualified to take advantage of or to enlarge the opportunities for participation. To them, participation is an innovation. The demand for participation in the continuing education of teachers should be suitable to their restricted abilities to perceive and exploit the chance for participation. They must be offered opportunities which are practical, obvious, and which take their interests into account.

Participation in the continuing education of teachers should be thought of as a political learning process that will instruct them about the opportunities for participation in the educational system as well as in other political areas. Therefore, a participation-oriented continuing education must be made politically possible, and its existence must be institutionally ensured in West Germany.

If participation is demanded in the continuing education of teachers so that they can influence innovations, the decision-making structures must actually meet the demand.

Decisions about the subject matter and the organization of work in the continuing education of teachers must be made by all parties involved.

Participation in the continuing education of teachers should provide not only for the increasing qualification to participate in decisions concerning the policy of education, but also for their inclusion in the process of the development of a curriculum. The possibility of providing opportunities for input into curriculum development within individual schools should be taken into account, for such opportunities could offer the teachers a means of direct influence over matters in which they are practically interested.(3)

When teachers are confronted with participation models which they have not conceived themselves, the resultant participation is often merely superficial, for such models cannot fully take into account the experiences and interests of the teachers. Therefore, processes of participation should be designed by the participants themselves.

In some federal states, various research projects provide the teachers with some opportunities for participation and to provide adequate institutionalization of these opportunities. It remains to be seen whether these efforts will act as models for further development.

NOTES

(1)   Jurgen Baumert and Jurgen Raschert, "Partizipation an curricularen Entscheidungsprozessen. Vorbereitung der Berliner Mittelstufenzentren durch praxisnahe Curriculum-entwicklung und Lehrerfortbildung," Zeitschrift fur Padagogik, 20 (1974), pp. 887-912

(2)   Reimer Gronemeyer, Integration durch Partizipation? (Frankfurt/Main, Arbeitsplatz/Wohnbereich: Fallstudien, 1973), p. 11

(3)   Raimund Klauser, Curriculumentwicklung in der Schule. Chancen zur Bewaltigung curricularer Innovationspraxis." Eckhard Steur and Walter Tenfelde, ed., Schulleitungs-ausbildung: Auf dem Wege zur innovativen Schule (Op-laden, 1978), pp. 117-127.

10 The Possibilities and Limits of Participation in North Rhine Westphalia's **Oberstufen-Kolleg** of the University of Bielefeld

Wulf Drexler

PRELIMINARY REMARKS

This study examines the Oberstufen-Kolleg (OS), an unprecedented educational institution which resembles in many respects the American college(1) and is the first and only German "college." Because it is part of the University of Bielefeld but is not subject to the normal rules and regulations governing German schools (the Regelschulsystem), the OS has been able to introduce innovations normally impossible in the Federal Republic. The educational goal of the OS is to close the gap between theoreticians and practitioners, which is particularly wide in the Federal Republic. This attempt is being made through the use of "action research," a research design which relies not only on the classical tools of empiricism but also on the participation of students and a large amount of feedback.(2) To achieve more real equality of opportunity than exists in the traditional three-class Regelschulsystem (Volks- or- Hauptschule) for the lower classes, Realschule for the middle classes, Gymnasium for the middle and upper classes), students and teachers are selected according to criteria which provide class balance. The OS has introduced other innovations as well, such as alternative systems for evaluating achievement and a diversified system of counseling. The OS has been under considerable outside pressure since its opening to students in the autumn of 1974. In addition to the limits placed on the OS by German institutions, there are characteristic German mechanisms that prevent innovations in organizations. These "external barriers to democratization and participation of German societal institutions" in many ways constrain the internal possibilities for participation and innovative change in an institution.

123

These mechanisms of immobility are the result of the special close-knit bureaucratic organization in the field of education which allows no exceptions whatsoever to standard methods.

The OS has also faced the opposition of large groups of German society that have vested interests in abolishing the OS because of its innovations, which make it markedly different from the rest of the traditional, very authoritarian German school system. As a result, the OS has suffered a number of defeats. The standing committee of all eleven state Ministers for Culture and Education (Kultusministerkonferenz) have taken the position that no experiments can be carried out, especially not ones concerning the Gymnasium, in part because of the present crisis in the strictly regulated area of university admissions. The OS was turned down by this committee, especially by the Bavarians, without even having the opportunity to present its own case. Ministry officials issued numerous erlasse (decrees that are binding on all civil servants they address) that the OS rejected in an unprecedented step. Subministerial intermediary-school governing authorities for Gymnasium then attempted to assume control of OS teacher recruitment.

The prospects for the OS are not encouraging. It has become nearly impossible for the OS to resist a further dismantling. First, the Ministry for Culture and Education has recently made its own man head of the OS. Second, the OS has lost its political support. The FDP has oriented its policy more toward the CDU, especially in the field of education, for it is likely to become the coalition partner of the CDU in the eighties. To counteract this trend, the SPD is not doing anything significant that is not in line with the other parties' lines. Although none of the three leading parties has openly attacked the OS, they distrust the OS increasingly because it is an institution difficult to assess and to control. Their attitude is justified because the OS continues to incite the public, even by acts of disobedience. The only positive development is the "Participation Law of 1978" (Schulmitwirkungesgesetz), which encourages participation possibilities for middle- and upper-class parents. It also grants to the Regelschulsystem more reliable openings for participation than the former ones, which were based on participation decrees which could be changed without notice.

The easiest solution for this recently formed grand coalition of politicians and administrators is to limit the internal freedom of decision of the OS by widening the 1978 law to regular participation in the Regelschulsystem. This loss of freedom to reorganize the institution will have severe repercussions for the curriculum and internal organization.

A BRIEF HISTORY OF THE OS

The background of the OS provides an explanation for this pessimism. The conditions in which the OS developed no longer exist. During the sixties, a high degree of consensus existed among elites about social innovations from above, especially in education. This attitude was a consequence of several factors. First, the Erhard economic policy of the early sixties, which sought the development of a highly competitive German industry, increased the demand for highly trained personnel. Second, the educational system, which had not changed much since Hitler, needed significant revision in order to increase the number of students in higher education. Third, a rising birth rate increased the demand for teachers. Finally, German conservatives, deeply concerned about the Cold War, were shocked into accepting a certain amount of educational change by the appearance of the first Sputnik.

The beginnings of the OS in this changing German climate can be traced to 1963, to the concepts of Hartmut von Hentig, one of the few educators who could formulate a new educational policy after the Nazi persecution of nearly all social scientists. Von Hentig, the initiator of the OS and the Laborschule, developed his concepts while at the University of Chicago and Gottingen and while a teacher of Latin and Greek in Germany.

The OS and the Laborschule were included in a newly founded "reform university" at Bielefeld in 1968 as a result of a decision by Mikat (CDU), the Minister for Culture and Education of NRW. That such a step was taken without reference to an act of parliament suggests that the decision makers were unaware of the radical practical consequences of von Hentig's educational theories. The elite were no doubt assured enough by von Hentig's strong reputation to place the reform in his hands. Thus, although they probably were never reviewed by the administration and the political elite, the educational theories of von Hentig were tacitly understood to be the framework for all further planning and were institutionalized directly under the gaze of the Ministry for Culture and Education and the Ministry for Research and Science. Although each ministry had a seat on a supervisory board, neither attempted to become involved in conceptual questions. The importance of von Hentig to the foundation of the OS cannot be underestimated.

The years 1970-1974 were a period of planning for the OS and Laborschule. Official planners, many of whom had been actively involved in the student movements and had had some experience in self-organization, were recruited, and they planned the curriculum, designed the building, and chose equipment.(3) Three of the four years were financed by the VW Foundation; the state of NRW took over financing in the fourth year after being reminded of its commitment by intensive lobbying by von Hentig and his staff.

The planning of the curriculum and its institutionalization proceeded without serious outside interference because of the support of the VW Foundation, the protection of the university, and the tacit consent of the ministries involved. However, when confronted with a lengthy, detailed proposal immediately before the opening of the school, the administrators and politicians withdrew their support, but they could not stop the implementation of the curriculum. After extensive internal debate, the school staff refused to compromise, and they opened the schools with administrators or politicians present. Even so, the OS still succeeded in placing a large number of staff positions in the budget in 1976 with the help of parliament and the state cabinet.

The major problems of the OS have been reduced to six, and there has been limited success in treating one of those. Acceptable agreements for admission of OS students to higher semesters at the university have been reached for all areas except law and medicine. The staff was forced to compromise on issues of confidential reports on teachers by governing authorities of the Gymnasium and final examinations. As for self-administration, the OS must deal with a state commissioner. The OS curriculum and the special admission criteria will probably be rejected by the Ministers for Culture and Education in 1980. After these defeats, what will remain, apart from the building and a highly committed personnel, is a Gymnasium that provides more students with admission to higher semesters of the university than the traditional one and that is permitted to do curriculum research within a narrow and highly controlled framework.

THE ORGANIZATIONAL MODEL OF SELF-ADMINISTRATION

The realization of von Hentig's educational idea of a free school as a scientific alternative to the Gymnasium and to the introductory education of the university necessarily called for new forms of participation and flexible, loosely knit organizational structures that allowed for the continuous changes and transformations dictated by new experience.

In retrospect, it is a great credit to von Hentig and his first staff members that they established a number of prerequisites for the later model of participation. First, decisions were made on a strictly democratic basis. Everyone was included in the decision-making process, including non-staff members such as typists. This was significant because there were very few opportunities to experience and practice democratic forms of participation in Germany before

the sixties. Second, a very careful recruitment policy
provided for a highly cooperative new staff. As a result,
those selected had the feeling of being accepted by everybody.
Third, several attempts were made to increase individual
participation by trying to reduce informal hierarchies, "bogus
authorities," and the importance of formal positions. The
intention of these measures was to find more soundly
established methods of creating consensus based on common
interests. Fourth, the planning staff formulated an internal
constitution based on widespread consensus that was later
passed by the "General Assembly" of the OS. It contained all
the important educational and institutional aims of the OS such
as the provision of tertiary education, student-centered
learning, curriculum research, and self-administration. This
constitution became very important for decision making after
the OS opened. Fifth, the planning staff developed a
functioning organizational structure to start self-administration
(Satzung) with students and parents.

   Presuppositions for this self-administration were developed
by a special committee set up in February 1973. This
committee studied historical development of participation in
schools and considered different proposals for participation and
their legal implications. It then sought a compromise between
the status quo in the Regelschulsystem and a "democratic
utopia" that was called a "realizable utopia" (Realutopie). To
defend the concept of decision making against restricting legal
concepts, they had to derive their own interpretation of
democracy from the Constitution of the Federal Republic.
While the limiting legal concepts were mainly based on
administrative interest in an efficient bureaucratic organization
of schools and on their educational aims, OS's considerations
were focused on constitutionally guaranteed basic rights of
parents, teachers and students.(4)

   As a result of these considerations, the following model of
decision making was constructed. All members of the OS,
including teachers, parents, students, administrators, and
typists, can take part in decision making. All meetings are
open to the internal public - including parents - except for
those concerned with confidential matters. The total number
of votes in the making of decisions is distributed among the
different groups according to their objective interests in the
particular decision being made. This distribution should be
determined by argument. Direct and indirect democratic
procedures are understood to be compatible and complementary
to one another. All work in institutionalized decision-making
bodies should be rewarded. Lower teaching assignments must
be given to staff members; equivalents of general education
courses must be provided for students; working time must be
allowed to administrators. To guarantee equal opportunities
for participation in decision making, all persons holding office

should be elected at regular intervals. To guarantee an equal division of work in self-administration, teachers must work on either a decision-making body or one of the 23 permanent committees which perform administrative tasks. They are also to work out proposals for the decision-making bodies to consider. All binding outside restrictions should be strictly observed. Among the relevant restrictions are that teachers must have at least 50 percent of all seats in all decision-making bodies (by decision of the Federal Constitution Court); that the OS is simultaneously a research institute of the University of Bielefeld as well as a college and a school (schools and universities are governed by different laws and regulations); and that representatives are only bound by their consciences.

The final draft of the plan was ratified unanimously by the Senat of the University of Bielefeld in June 1974. However, it was rejected by the ministries. In February 1977, a new draft, which incorporated several changes made because of the objections of the ministries, was ratified by the University but again rejected by the ministries. Thus, since 1974, OS has been in the precarious situation of having to work without any approved regulations. This situation has had advantages, however. It has created an opportunity to experiment with the original concept of self-administration. Also, the scope for self-administration has been broadened. Because the Academic Advisory Board, created as a link between the University and OS, could not be installed, its duties had to be assumed by other decision-making bodies.

It was also proposed that the school head and his deputy be elected and confirmed in office with the consent of the ministries for a term of four years. However, this procedure was unacceptable to the Ministry for Culture and Education and to the state and federal Ministry of Interior (both headed by FDP ministers) because headmasters must be appointed for life according to well-established civil service regulations. As a result, OS was never run with an officially approved headmaster. Instead of a headmaster, a so-called spokesman was elected yearly.

Aside from these modifications, the model of self-administration describes how the OS has worked for four-and-one-half years. The headmaster, or spokesman, and his deputy are in charge of that part of the OS which is the school and cooperate closely with the Conference. Advising and assisting the headmaster, the Conference decides on questions concerning the OS as a school, such as the admission of students, time tables, personal requests, the budget, and house rules. The Curriculum Council itself decides upon questions of curriculum research and guidelines for curricula and, along with the Conference, is responsible for the recruitment of new staff members. The Convention, or

General Assembly, decides upon basic questions concerning the OS as a whole, such as the total curriculum, institutional and educational aims, self-administration, and conflicts between decision-making bodies. It elects the headmaster, his deputy, and the deputy to the administrative head of Curriculum Research, Hartmut von Hentig. The head of Curriculum Research and his deputy (Wissenschaftliche Leitung) are in charge of all research questions outside of the scope of other decision-making bodies. They have to coordinate research programs and cooperate closely with the Curriculum Council.

A First Analysis of the Model of Self-Administration in Use Since Autumn 1974

The organizational model of self-administration described above gained its stability and its legitimacy without being officially approved and in spite of several adverse conditions. The students entering the OS had had little or no experience in democratic procedures. New members, having rights equal to those of the old members, had to be integrated. The OS opened in September 1974, with 218 students and 30 teachers, 20 of whom had worked on the planning of the project and thus formed the core of the new teaching staff. It grew to 800 students and 80 staff members by September 1978. Permanent, outside pressures and insecurity made continuous work impossible and, even worse, used up about one-fourth of the teachers' time, which was urgently needed for the development of curricula, especially in medicine, that would be acceptable to students and university departments.

The organizational model was accepted by almost everybody primarily because of the following reasons.

The OS was highly integrative. New teachers and students accepted the OS, partly out of self-interest. Teachers wanted to keep their new status as something between a school teacher and a university teacher. Students saw themselves no longer as pupils, but as part of the university. In part, they accepted the OS because they could easily identify themselves with its educational and institutional aims. Common reactions to outside pressures enforced this process until the end of 1977, when it became evident that the battle was partly lost and that a major revision of the OS was necessary.

The teaching of self-administration and of self-determination was deeply rooted in the educational conception of von Hentig, and it was carried on in individual courses. The special organization of courses intensified the awareness of problems of self-administration and made participation accessible to everybody. In times of threat to the institution it was even possible to use regular courses to work out counterstrategies.

The efficiency of the daily administration of the OS was continuously increased by treating all recurrent routing decisions the same way, thus saving time for the discussion of other questions.

In comparison to other educational institutions, the OS was characterized by especially high involvement of its members. In critical situations this involvement naturally increased. For example, upon the arrival of the Informationserlass, almost 70 percent of all students and teachers went by bus to Dusseldorf to demonstrate in front of the ministries and to force them into a public discussion, even though they had been told by the Erlass to stay at home.

Decision making proved to be a highly flexible and unbureaucratic process. The method of decision making varied depending on the issue and on who or what body had taken the initiative. As a rule, important and urgent issues were first discussed in plenary sessions, then different propositions were worked out in small ad hoc groups and/or decision-making bodies. These propositions were discussed again in a plenary session before the final decision was made by the responsible body, frequently the General Assembly. In most cases, plenary meetings and decision-making bodies worked hand in hand, especially in times when speedy decisions had to be made on complex problems.

In critical situations the OS was able to mobilize its own resources and thus was partly successful in counteracting Erlasse of the ministries. The OS managed to put numerous pressures on the ministries through a demonstration and a two-week active strike by students, a project called "Save the OS," which was worked on instead of regular courses, and an open letter from parents, students, and teachers.

The organizational model of self-administration of the OS has worked astonishingly well in spite of many adverse factors and many problems still to be solved. The OS was certainly the first German school to develop and to put into effect a practicable model for participation. It also shows that countries like the Federal Republic do possess the conceptual, personal, and financial resources to create new educational institutions that could cope much better with the interests, needs, and problems of present-day students, parents, and teachers.

INTERNAL BARRIERS TO PARTICIPATION AND
QUESTIONS FOR FURTHER RESEARCH

As the case of the OS demonstrates, the external barriers to participation in education in the Federal Republic are extremely high, and can be removed only through joint endeavors of many societal groups. These restrictions lead to many latent and manifest repercussions for the quality of learning and for the ability of the individual to participate in school and in society at large. In a closely knit bureaucratic and judicial system, nobody takes personal responsibility, which is replaced by an abstract, legalistic, and hierarchical system in which there is circular responsibility and issues are passed from one person to another like a hot potato. The resulting quality of participation can be illustrated by examination of the "hidden curriculum" of the Regelschulsystem, for which the OS tried to find an alternative. In the "hidden curriculum," one learns to depend on uncontrollable and anonymous powers against which nothing can be done. Also, one adjusts to the rituals and rules of the school without recognizing and comprehending their functions. One may learn that grading is not based solely on personal progress in learning but also on adjustment to superiors and on the maneuvering of fellow students. Creativity, spontaneity, openness of mind, and critical ability (except for criticism of out-groups) are often suspect. One can learn the fear of failing and thereby become a worthless person.

In order to transform a school from a highly regulated system into an institution that fosters autonomy and self-determination, one has to both experiment and relax the system. This process often leads to a too high degree of permissiveness, which has a negative effect, particularly on those students not yet used to continuous work and personal freedom. The outside pressures reinforce this behavior because they require time and energy and internal solidarity to counteract. Many members of the OS feel that internal solidarity should not be threatened by too serious internal conflicts now. Thus, important conflicts remain latent, and major revisions of the original educational conceptions on the basis of past experience have not yet been made.

The quality of participation within an institution is determined to a large extent by factors such as the initial levels of participation of new members; by the organizational structure of decision making (whether it is strictly regulated or more open); by the choice of teaching methods (whether authoritarian, laissez-faire, student-oriented, etc.); by the level of participation achieved by old members; and by the institution's ability to integrate different interests and levels of participation through common aims. These factors are interdependent. For example, an authoritarian teaching method is usually paralleled by a rigid organizational structure and insufficient ability of individuals to participate. Thus, at the OS there is good reason to believe that the interplay among self-administration, student-oriented teaching, action research, and common institutional and educational aims will eventually increase the ability to transfer processes of learning

and decision making to individuals. It will also make possible
more cooperation with new members, providing them with a
better start for their own development. This interplay should
lead to behavioral changes. Because such an institutional
arrangement grants individuals important rights, they learn to
identify with them and gain new insights by using them
successfully. Among the preconditions for the learning of
participation (not all of which have been realized at the OS, as
discussed above), are that individuals must have genuine
alternatives available in their decision making. They must
know that the decision to vote for an alternative is legitimate
and is the exercise of an inalienable right. In addition to
knowing the whole range of alternatives open to them,
individuals should know the procedures for legitimizing new
alternatives. They should have the feeling that decision
making and learning are organized and accomplished by people
and are based on consensus about long-term institutional and
educational aims, on mutual trust and reliability, and on an
active protection of minorities. The individuals should be
aware of major developments outside the institution which may
have important internal repercussions or may help in finding a
common basis for a realizable balance between internal and
external demands. Finally, they should realize through their
own experience that to increase everybody's quality of
participation is a difficult and life-long process of learning
that depends more on behavioral change than on intellectual
insight; they should also realize that this personal learning
process affects societal developments by affecting the way
people meet and deal with deep personal and societal
contradictions, which generally can be removed by only the
joint effort of many persons.

It is difficult to say to what extent the OS has thus far
increased the quality of participation of its members in
comparison to that of the Regelschulsystem. Detailed empirical
research and criteria for different qualities or levels of
participation are required for such an evaluation.

The following definitions of levels of participation are
suggested by the work of Kohlberg, who developed five levels
of moral judgments. The participation levels, however, are
concerned more with behavioral than cognitive development.
Although little research has been done so far in the area of
quantifying or qualifying participation, these levels may be
helpful in beginning that work. The specific examples for
each level are drawn from the experience of OS participants.

First level of participation: dependence on uncontrollable,
irrational, and anonymous powers.

At this level, one's own actions are mainly directed by
obedience and the fear of punishment. In the absence of

uncontrollable powers, one wastes time and is not motivated to do anything meaningful. One attends courses intermittently and forgets the work one wanted to do or promised to do.

Second level: naive, egoistic orientation.

Students on this level are not interested in democracy or participation. They want an academic job with a minimum of costs and a maximum of benefits. They can be helped to find out more about their needs by means of experience and with the use of scientific methods and findings.

Third level: conformity to conventions and norms; orientation toward the ideal of the "good boy" and the "nice girl."

At this level, one tries to help and to please others. In case of conflict, one sticks with the majority and attempts to avoid trouble. For this one is willing to defer one's own needs. Students at this level work in a responsible way but do not want to expose and commit themselves. Through positive experience with the institution and because of student-centered learning, they increasingly identify with the institution and begin to defend their own experiences and the newly acquired knowledge and abilities.

Fourth level: legalistic orientation toward contracts.

Here, common rules and expectations are seen as a starting point for agreements. Although some of the rules are arbitrary, once a contract is signed it has to be kept. (Many decisions of the Curriculum Council were made on this basis, sometimes to the disadvantage of specific cases.)

Fifth level: orientation toward universal principles.

At this highest level orientation is not based on specific interests, such as class, sex, religious affiliation, nationality, etc., but rather on principles which are universal and consistent.

NOTES

(1) Publications about the Oberstufen-Kolleg (selection): H. v. Hentig et al., Das Bielefelder Oberstufen-Kolleg (Stuttgart, 1971); H. v. Hentig, Schule als Erfahrungsraum? (Stuttgart: Klett Verlag, 1974); W. Harder, Drei Jahre Curriculum-Werkstatten (Stuttgart: Klett Verlag, 1974); Ausbildungsgange am Oberstufen-Kolleg

des Landes NRW an der Universitat Bielefeld, Vorlage an
das Kultusministerium, Marz 1974; Schriftenreihe der
Schulprojekte Laborschule/Oberstufen-Kolleg im Klett
Verlag; AMBOS, Arbeitsmaterialien aus dem Oberstufen-
Kolleg, Bielefeld.

(2) See also W. Drexler and G. Wenzel-Glassing "Curriculumentwicklung und Handlungsforschung," Bielefeld,
1976 (unpublished paper).

(3) The Laborschule encompasses the primary stage,
including one preschool year, and 11 grades of the
secondary stage; this means that pupils are taught there
from the ages of five to sixteen. The school is organized
along the lines of a fully integrated, comprehensive
school, with classes lasting the whole day, and has place
for 660 pupils. The Laborschule and Obserstufen-Kolleg
belong together as curriculum workshops, since both were
planned by the same staff. Many problems I want to
outline here are equally applicable to the situation of the
Laborschule.

(4) See L. Dietze, "Schulverfassung und Grundgesetz,
Demokratieprinzip und Mitbestimmung in der Schulreform,"
Jur. Diss. (1972).

IV
Urban Policy

11 Citizens' Participation in the Delivery of Human Services
Gordon P. Whitaker

Citizen participation has been viewed as both a means and an end. Some have considered increased citizen participation primarily as a mechanism for improving the quality of public policy - for making the distribution of public services more equitable and the content of public services more responsive to the needs and desires of people in general, and the poor and disadvantaged in particular. Others have been concerned about improving the participation of citizens for itself, believing that the very experience of self-government is valuable for human beings.[1] Regardless of emphasis, however, there is general agreement that the participation of citizens refers to actions intended to influence. Usually the actions thought of as constituting citizens' participation include voting, campaigning, testifying, petitioning, lobbying, and other explicit efforts to influence policy decisions. The focus has usually been on changing laws or regulations or budgets or personnel. There is, though, another aspect of citizens' participation which requires attention.

Citizens influence the content of many public services through their direct participation in service delivery. This is especially the case for human services - activities designed to change people directly rather than to change their physical environment. Most economic activity, including that of many public agencies, is directed toward the production of goods. Raw materials are transformed into products which can then be delivered to consumers. Human services are not like that. Education or health care or crisis intervention have as their primary objective the transformation of the consumer. Others may benefit from a child's education or a worker's good health or the pacification of a husband and wife, but the primary beneficiaries are the clients themselves. The concepts "raw material," "finished product," and "consumer" breakdown in

137

human services because all refer to the same individual.(2)   In
this context the term "delivery" takes on a new meaning, also.
The agent delivering human services is much like the doctor or
midwife delivering a baby.   The agent uses his or her skills
and   conducts   activities   to   facilitate   the   process.   But   the
person being served also has a major responsibility for the
service.(3)
     The   analogy   between   the   delivery   of   babies   and   the
delivery of human services generally is further instructive if
we look at the recent history of childbirth practices in the
United States.   For a number of years, the accepted view of
childbirth held that it was a medical procedure in which the
pregnant   woman   was   a   passive   patient   to   her   doctor's
ministrations.   Even at her most sedated and least regarded,
however, the woman played a vital part in the baby's birth.
In the past few years, a broader recognition of the importance
of prenatal care and a reassertion by many women of their role
in childbirth has brought about a change in the way doctors
treat their pregnant patients.   Proponents of increased mother
participation argue that it is both a means to healthier babies
and an important end in itself for the women who experience
it.   So it is for all human services.

CITIZENS AS COPRODUCERS

Because "delivery" of services so strongly connotes conveyance
of an already finished product to someone who will use it, an
alternative   term   may   be   preferable.   Perhaps   it   would   be
helpful to use the phrase "coproduction" of human services.
For in human services the agent helps the person being served
to make the desired sorts of changes.   Whether it is learning
new   ideas   or   new   skills,   acquiring   healthier   habits,   or
changing one's outlook on family or society, only the individual
served can accomplish the change.   He or she is a vital
coproducer of any personal transformation that occurs.   The
agent can supply encouragements, suggest options, illustrate
techniques, and provide guidance and advice, but the agent
alone cannot bring about the change.   Instead of the agent
delivering a service to the citizen, agent and citizen coproduce
the service.
     The notion of citizens as coproducers of public services is
certainly at variance with common ideas of how governments
operate and how services are produced.   A brief review of
some recent discussions of citizens' participation will illustrate
this point.   As with any modish term, "citizens' participation"
has been used in a variety of ways.
     One   use   of   the   term   is   to   indicate   the   lobbying
and litigation efforts of "public interest groups and citizen

organizations."(4)   This usage refers not to the activities of individual citizens so much as to the representation of

> broad public needs and interests as distinct from the more narrow, private, largely economic interests rep-resented by trade association, labor unions, ethnic groups, and other traditional interest groups.(5)

In his discussion of the participation of citizens, Cupps is concerned with the influence such groups have on the formulation of policy through their effects on rule making in the courts, the legislature, and, particularly, the administrative agencies of the federal government. While Cupps recognizes that administrative agencies as well as "political" institutions make policy and can be subject to lobbying, he does not discuss the possibility that citizens might influence the <u>execution</u> of public policy as well as its formulation.   He implicitly accepts the view of policy implementation as the mechanical carrying out of decisions made by a "higher authority."   Cupps is also primarily concerned with the policy views being expressed and not with the generality of their expression.   He is interested in how the concerns of traditionally less influential parts of the populace are now being expressed to federal policy makers.   Even though that expression is indirect, through representatives, Cupps refers to the phenomenon as "citizens' participation."

A generally similar use of "citizens' participation" refers to the representation of neighborhood or ethnic group interests in local policy making.   During the past fifteen years many cities have instituted programs in which citizens can participate, at least partly in response to federal grants-in-aid requirements.   While some of these consist of nothing more than a few public hearings, more elaborate programs are common.   Many in fact constitute adjunct public authorities or representative bodies.   In the Community Action Program model, a not-for-profit corporation is created to receive public funds and administer programs under the authority of a council of citizens.   In the Urban Renewal model, a citizens' advisory board is formed to review government plans for specific types of public programs in target areas.   In both cases, participation by citizens at large is seen as attending public hearings, electing representatives, and expressing opinions to and through those representatives.   Thus discussion of citizens' participation programs in cities, like the programs themselves, usually focus on the activities of the representatives rather than those of citizens generally.(6)

The aspect of large-scale participation of citizens which has received the most attention from political scientists in the United States is voting, but in the past decade-and-a-half other citizens' activities which influence decision makers have been studied. Verba and Nie, for example, include as citizens' participation twelve types of activity, only two of which are voting. Greenberg considers a similar set of activities, adding only violence as another way for citizens to influence public policy.(7)

In these studies, the central concern is to find ways in which citizens attempt to influence the policy decisions of public officials, not the execution of public policy. Almond and Verba express this distinction as the difference between a person's activities as "citizen" and that same person's activities as "subject":

> The competent citizen has a role in the formation of general policy. Furthermore, he plays an <u>influential</u> role in this decision-making process: he participates by using explicit or implicit threats of some form of deprivation if the official does not comply with his demand. The subject does not participate in making rules, nor does his participation involve the use of political influence. His participation comes at the point at which general policy has been made and is being applied.(8)

In such a view, government may be democratic, but administration is not. Administration is seen as technical and, therefore, neutral.

Almond and Verba express a common point of view when they distinguish between an "upward flow of policy making" through which citizens exercise influence and a "downward flow of policy enforcement" toward which the citizen has "essentially a passive relationship."(9) The distinction has some force, of course. Examples abound of public policies that are carried out without the cooperation of the general citizenry. The United States space program is a good illustration. Once policy was approved and funds allocated, experts took over and produced and deployed the machinery. But it is dangerous that we run programs such as public education in the same way. The pupil and his or her parents, fully as much as the teacher, influence what education that pupil obtains. The best of lesson plans, instructional materials, and teaching techniques cannot educate the child who will not learn. Coproduction is essential for human service.

Ostrom has labeled our preoccupation with the distinction between politics and administration as the "Intellectual Crisis in American Public Administration."(10) He argues that in adopting Weber's ideas about hierarchical control and Wilson's ideas about a single locus of decision making, we have come to expect the behavior of bureaucrats to be determined. In fact, the actions of the "street-level bureaucrat," especially in human services, are far from determined. Lipsky points this out and offers an example:

> Consider the rookie policeman who, in addition to responding to his own conceptions of the policeman's role, must accommodate the demands placed upon him by (1) fellow officers in the station house who teach him how to get along and try to correct the teachings of his police academy instructors; (2) his immediate superiors who may strive for efficiency at the expense of current practices; (3) police executives who communicate expectations contradictory to station house mores; and (4) the general public, who in American cities today is likely to be divided along both class and racial lines in its expectations of police practices and behavior. (11)

Ostrom suggests that we should view all public employees and all citizens as decision makers when regarding the public services with which they deal. Laws and rules in such a system should not be seen as prescribing a specific course of action. Rather they are constraints within which people make decisions. Laws and regulations are statements of the likely consequences of taking certain courses of action. As such, they serve as benchmarks against which one assesses the wisdom of alternatives, but they do not determine behavior; neither do orders prescribe specific acts. Interpretation and interpolation are commonplace. (12) In large measure public business is conducted in this way, but this is rarely acknowledged. The importance of the knowledge and judgment of "street-level" public employees and the citizens they serve is ignored.

Many public services require for their execution the active involvement of members of the general public and, especially, of those who are to be the direct beneficiaries of the service. In a strict sense, not even the formal status of "citizen" is required for these sorts of participation. In most cases, any member of the community, regardless of age or residency or nationality, may participate in human services in the United States.

TYPES OF COPRODUCTION

Three broad types of activities constitute coproduction: citizens requesting assistance from public agents; citizens providing assistance to public agents; and citizens and agents interacting to mutually adjust service expectations and actions. (13)

Many public service activities are carried out only in response to specific requests from citizens. Social security, welfare, unemployment, and medicare payments all depend on citizens applying. Emergency assistance from fire, police, or medical personnel is usually initiated by citizens' request. The extent to which citizens who need these services receive them depends largely upon the extent to which they (or their neighbors) request assistance. Not only human services are subject to this type of influence by citizens. A number of public agencies that produce changes in the physical environment are organized to respond primarily to problems identified by concerned citizens.

The point seems obvious. Yet only in the past few years have many public agencies begun to conduct "outreach" programs to inform citizens of the services they offer and to encourage those in need to apply. Similarly, only recently have agencies made efforts to facilitate the receipt and processing of unusual service requests. This is not surprising given our common view of the responsibilities of public employees: that the work of the service agent is closely circumscribed by administrative rules and procedures. The agent's use of personal knowledge or judgment is precluded. Decision making at that level is limited to sorting cases into appropriate categories. Katz and his colleagues describe the model procedure, not unapprovingly, this way:

> On one side of the desk sits the applicant for service, with all the needs, experiences, and idiosyncratic characteristics that combined to bring him there. On the other side of the desk sits a person whose function it is to determine the validity of the presenting request, the goodness of fit between it and the franchise of the agency, and thus the entitlement of the person. It is likely to be a brief conversation, although the preliminaries may be long. It ends with a decision, or a referral, either of which may satisfy or frustrate the client.(14)

When the circumstances and requests do not fit this model, as they often do not for teachers, police officers, and other human service agents, public agents may find themselves with no guidance to follow. Unless these agents have been encouraged to develop and to use their judgment, informally defined categories of people and problems based on personal experiences and prejudices and the views of peers, frequently replace administrative regulations as the categories for sorting cases.(15)

A central issue is who defines "need." How much credence are service agents prepared to place in a citizen's description of problems and needs when that description differs from the agency's definition? Many requests for emergency police assistance, for example, concern family arguments and fights. Standard police response has been to separate the parties from the argument and to get one of them to leave the scene if possible. Because police have usually defined their work as "crime fighting," domestic disturbance calls have commonly been viewed by officers as nuisances, although the danger they can pose is widely recognized. Where such calls are considered as outside the scope of "real police work," little training is given to officers in appropriate skills for handling these situations and little attention is directed to evaluating how well officers deal with them. Many departments do not even keep accounts of the number of calls of this type they receive, although they keep detailed records on calls they are interested in - reports of crime. The situation is changing, however. Some police departments are beginning to examine the kinds of service requests they receive in order to train their officers with skills appropriate for those problems, and to find out how well their officers deal with them.(16)

Thus, official recognition of what is requested by citizens has led some agencies to revise their training and supervision practices. But this has not meant simply the introduction of a new set of standard operating procedures for family crisis intervention. Instead, it has often involved a redefinition of the police officer's role. Training for intervening in a crisis involves development of each officer's powers of discernment and judgment. It encourages the officer to view disputants not as cases to be categorized and responded to as types, but to examine each problem situation and respond to the problems the disputants themselves are presenting.(17)

Citizens' requests for service may also influence the distribution of service allocations in a community. Some agencies may serve only those who make bureaucratically acceptable requests. For example, a library with a stock of books appealing only to highly educated readers with traditional tastes will continue to circulate books among only those readers so long as new book orders reflect past patterns of usage. To reach new readers from other cultural backgrounds, the library staff must learn which books (and other media) appeal to nonusers.(18)

Encouraging people to request new or different service activities may seem unwise for communities with scarce public resources. But in cases where the activities being conducted by public employees are seldom used (or used by only a small, comparatively well-to-do part of the community) continuation of current service activities results in ineffective or inequitable public policies. Especially in places where the residents (and their tastes, circumstances, and behaviors) are changing, agencies which rely on citizens' requests for services need to be alert to (and help to encourage) requests for assistance with new types of problems. Unless public service agents are also encouraged to recognize and respond appropriately to new types of service requests, their actions are not likely to be as helpful as they could and should be.

Not every agency can be equipped to handle every problem, of course. In many instances, referral to another agency may be the most appropriate response. To make good referrals, service agents need accurate information about other service agencies: referral should also be viewed as a service. Moreover, some requests will be for special treatment or favors which cannot be provided because they constitute unfair privileges or a failure to enforce rights and duties. Agents must be responsible to the law and to considerations of equity as well as to the particular requests of individuals. Each public servant accepts a substantial public trust and must be held accountable for his or her use of that responsibility.

Coproduction by citizens of public services through service requests is not an adversarial form of participation. Although it is possible for citizens to overload an agency with requests or to boycott an agency in order to force some policy change, that is not the kind of influence which is most pervasive. There is a continual shaping of what an agency does by the kinds of requests made on it by citizens. Citizens' requests for service are the operational definition of objectives for most human service and some other public agencies. Recognition of agency dependence on service requests and citizens' problems in communicating requests in agency terms is important to improve this form of citizen participation in service delivery.

The success of many public policies depends upon the behavior of the citizenry. For human services, the transformation of citizens' behavior is the immediate service objective. Too often that point is overlooked. The police officer who stops a reckless driver may view the act as apprehensive of a violator of the law. A more constructive view of that interaction is that the officer is attempting to change the driver's behavior to reduce the likelihood that the driver will injure himself or others. This latter point of view is more constructive because officers who hold it are apt to focus their attention on drivers whose behavior is dangerous, while those who hold the "law enforcement" view may devote attention to less hazardous infractions which are commonly more numerous.

The behavior of citizens whose actions are not the target of agency concern also often influences the execution of public policy. The importance of parents' actions in the education of their children is one example. Another is the role residents and other users of an area play in maintaining public safety in

the area.   Fifteen years ago when Jacobs wrote that through
certain kinds of routine daily behavior toward their neighbors
people could prevent burglaries and street crimes, her analysis
was viewed as highly novel.(19)   Today the major textbook for
police administrators takes the position that "if there are no
effective forces of community social control at work, there is
little if anything the police can do to deal with crime and
lawlessness."(20)   The social disintegration of neighborhoods
and changes in expectations about how to relate to neighbors
have left many places without the kind of shared concern for
the common welfare that supports public safety.   Thus, actions
which assist police, such as neighbors watching each others'
property,   no   longer   occur   as   a   part   of   routine   social
interaction.   In the absence of such behavior, police have
begun   to   encourage   it   through   special   crime-prevention
programs.(21)   General citizen cooperation in public programs
becomes increasingly important with the continued weakening of
the family and small-group relationships through which people
used to work for common goals. Cooperation with public agents
in pursuit of a common objective is an important form of
political participation.

Cooperation needs to be distinguished from compliance and
habit, of course.   If citizens act in accord with public service
goals because they fear reprisals for their refusal, or if
citizens act in accord with public goals because they have
become habituated to that set of behaviors, their actions do
not constitute cooperation.   Cooperation is voluntary.   The
potential for influence by citizens on public service through
"assistance" depends upon the capacity to withhold or to give
cooperation.   Similarly   the   contributions   of   cooperation   to
individuals' citizenship in a democracy depend upon their
perceiving a choice and their weighing the personal and public
consequences of participating.

Opportunities   for   citizens'   cooperation   are   thus   also
opportunities for noncooperation.   Noncooperation can have as
powerful an influence on public services as cooperation.   One
situation in which citizens' cooperation (or noncooperation) is
especially influential is the introduction of a new public program requiring widespread citizens' activity.   The program
need not even be a human service.   An example is the recent
attempt of several cities to institute curb-side garbage pickup
for residents who have been accustomed to back-door pickup.
Facing revenue limits, a number of cities have sought to
reduce the costs of garbage collection by shifting some of the
labor from city employees to residents.   By having residents
place their garbage cans at the curb on collection days, the
cities could collect the same amount of garbage per truck in
the same (or less) time and reduce staff by one worker per
truck.   This would result in considerable savings of public
funds.   But citizens' cooperation is essential to this plan.
Compliance would be difficult to enforce - the garbage must be

collected for maintenance of sanitation and public health, and fines for noncompliance would be unwieldy on a massive scale.

The distinction between cooperation and compliance is often hazy, because the enforceability of sanctions is always open to question in the courts. In the United States, those who do not comply with what they regard as unjust behavioral requirements of governments have increasingly turned to the courts for relief from sanctions. When the courts ruled that compliance with laws racially segregating public facilities was unenforceable in the United States, noncooperation with the old public policy of segregation soon changed the patterns of seating on buses and at lunchcounters in the South.(22) Citizen noncooperation - even in the face of possible sanctions - received a major impetus from the Civil Rights movement. Citizens increasingly influence public policy by their noncooperation whether it is recognized formally through court suits or, more commonly, through the acquiescence of public officials in the failures of citizens to comply.

One way for citizens to disagree with officials that a policy is good is to fail to cooperate. If enough citizens withhold their assistance, a project based on cooperation cannot succeed. As Washnis concludes:

> It appears that not much meaningful will ever be done about reducing crime without the active concern of all citizens. Responsible individual citizens will have to take the lead in setting up ways to get residents involved, and simultaneously police and other city officials will have to understand citizen involvement, encourage it, and provide some resources and incentives to keep it going.(23)

Citizens' cooperation can be used to influence explicit policy choices - laws, regulations, or program plans, for example. But like citizens' requests, cooperation also has a continual, day-to-day effect on the content of public policy and the citizenship of the people.

In some situations involving the delivery of public service, agents and citizens interact to establish a common understanding of the citizen's problem and what each of them can do to help deal with it. This reciprocal modification of expectations and actions involves more communication than a simple request for assistance. It also involves more than the citizen's acquiescence to or rejection of the action proposed by the service agent. Sometimes no agreement is reached on what needs to be done or how to do it, but mutual adjustment occurs when the actions taken by both the service agent and the citizen are based on their joint consideration of a problem.

Mutual adjustment is most important in the delivery of human services. Of course, mutual adjustment of expectations and behavior is not the only way to transform people's behavior. Both persuasion and coercion are also used. Gersuny and Rosengren discuss a number of manipulative techniques used by service agents to secure coproduction of human services. Their review of the rhetoric used by agencies (mainly private, profit making) to persuade the gullible to cooperate, suggests that too often citizens may be unwilling or unable to exercise independent judgment about their actions.(24) Although persuasion is by no means all fakery, their discussion illustrates the need for citizens to maintain a healthy skepticism about persuasive appeals. A healthy skepticism about public agents' use of coercion is also valuable in a democracy. But like persuasion, coercion also has its place in government. Police powers are necessary to "reduce the advantages which the remorseless and the strong have over the sensitive and the civilized."(25) Taxing powers are needed to enforce equitable distribution of the costs of public policy, and the power to select and remove officials is a necessary check on their exercise of power and position.(26)

While mutual adjustment is not possible in all situations of the delivery of public service, it seems clearly possible and preferable in many situations. In an exchange of this type, both the citizen and the agent share responsibility for deciding what action to take. Moreover, each accords legitimacy to the responsibility of the other. The citizen-coproducer is not a "client" in the sense that he or she is not a supplicant seeking the favor of the agent.

The importance of mutual adjustment between teacher and student is suggested by experiments which found that teachers' expectations of student achievement have a marked influence on how well students do at their studies.(27) Teachers who look for potential in their students are more likely to find the potential which the students have and to tailor their teaching to stimulate that potential. From the other side, students who see their teachers as capable of presenting materials of interest and importance to the students are likely to commit themselves more vigorously to their own education then are students who are simply expected to cooperate or forced to comply.(28)

Mutual adjustment is important in policing, too.(29) For example, Muir quotes an officer's account of his encounter with a young man who had armed himself with a bat to avenge his younger sister's rape:

> I took the guy with the bat into a small cubicle all by ourselves and appealed both to his pride and to his manhood. I told him honestly, if I was the object of his hostilities - I didn't say it quite this way, but this was the general idea - I wouldn't take off my badge and fight it out with him. He was too

big for me, and besides I would have to arrest him,
and no one wants to arrest him. He didn't do
anything wrong. I try to give everyone an avenue
of escape. You have got to save his face. Some
devices for that are privacy - he can walk out of
that cubicle just as big as he went in and as
strong as ever. But alone I could advise him to do
it the right way. Next day, get on a phone to the
police department, and get a policeman, or a juvenile
officer to come out to the house. And interview
him, his sister, his mother, his grandmothers. Get
statements, even do some medical testing on the
sister. He went for that eventually. Initially, you
see, he would have sacrificed himself, would have
gone to jail knowingly. But he had no alternatives
in mind; he had to beat up the guy who had raped
his little sister. So you have to offer an individual
an escape from his bind. But a policeman cannot
afford to lose, and what you have to avoid as a
policeman is putting yourself into a spot with a
win-or-lose basis. I could have presented an
ultimatum. "You shut up or you're going to jail."
The final ultimatum is the authority to arrest, and
there is a perfect legal right to do it. But is it
going to be a peace-keeping move - and especially in
the long run?(30)

The officer in this encounter is clearly trying to inform and
persuade the young man with the bat, but he is also listening
and shaping his own expectations and behavior on the basis of
the young man's explanations and the possibility of a
noncoercive resolution. Similarly, the young man was willing
to listen to the officer and consider his information and
advice.
    Mutual adjustment obviously does not involve the
interaction of equals. The service agent almost always has
greater resources. The agent generally has the advantage of
greater skill or special knowledge. This professional authority
normally gives the agent a socially accepted power to prescribe
actions for the service recipient.(31) Or the agent may have
special legal authority to use force or impose other sanctions.
But authority, either professional or legal, may be sufficient
to induce the kind of personal change which many problems of
citizens seem to demand. As Davis found in a study of
patients' compliance with doctors' advice:

Communication between doctor and patient ideally
necessitates a certain degree of reciprocity. Each
person has certain rights and obligations. When the
doctor performs a service, the patient is obliged to

> reciprocate: first, by cooperating with the doctor in
> their interaction; and second, by complying with the
> medical recommendation once he leaves the doctor's
> office. We have seen, however, that there are
> deviations from these norms.(32)

Patients who were overbearing tended to ignore the advice of
more passive physicians. Conversely, doctors who questioned
patients extensively, but failed to share their use of the
information with the patient were also less likely to be obeyed.
Davis concludes:

> In the doctor-patient relationship, whether in private
> practice, hospital clinic, or on a ward, the doctor
> must rely on his ability to establish good rapport in
> order to inculcate in his patient a positive
> orientation and commitment to the relationship so that
> ultimately the patient will follow his advice. In
> order to do this, it becomes necessary for the doctor
> continually to explore and diagnose the social and
> psychological facets of his interaction with his
> patients as well as the manifest medical problem.(33)

The agent does not relinquish professional or legal authority when engaging in mutual adjustment of expectations
and actions. Rather the agent helps the citizen being served
by sharing authority. Thus the doctor explains the diagnosis
and how alternative treatments might work and the police
officer explains the basis of actions and the legal options
available.

The importance of coproduction, and especially mutual
adjustment, to delivery of human services is presented vividly
in Norval Morris's analysis of the failure of convict
rehabilitation programs. Morris argues that the
diagnosis/treatment model which prescribes rehabilitative
activities for the inmate and obtains the inmate's compliance
with those activities has not been successful because it has
ignored the crucial role that motivation plays in shaping
behavior.(34) If an inmate participates in training programs
or counseling only because he knows that doing so will earn
him privileges in prison and perhaps reduce the time he must
spend there, we should not be surprised that the "training"
and "counseling" have little effect on his life once he has been
released. Unless they really want to change their lives, or at
least explore that option as an alternative, prisoners do not
really participate in rehabilitation programs; they just go
through the motions. Morris recommends that inmates who so
desire should be given professional assistance in learning how
to live within the law as citizens of a free society. No special
inducements, which in prison are simply the back side of
coercion, should be offered. The sentencing to prison is one

thing. Rehabilitation activities are another. In the long run,
even those over whom a democratic society exercises the
greatest control cannot be forced to change their personal
behavior. A prisoner's active, voluntary participation is
required for public agents to help facilitate that kind of
change.(35)

Mutual adjustment is not feasible in all service situations.
Sometimes public agents have to coerce some citizens - even at
the cost of foregoing the opportunity to help them - in order
to protect other citizens. For coproduction to be possible,
citizens, as well as agents, must be willing to recognize the
legitimacy of the public policies the agents are charged with
implementing. At the very least, they must be willing to talk
and listen. As Reiss notes, "a civil police depends upon a
civil citizenry."(36) Citizens' participation in the reciprocal
transformation of agent and citizens' expectations and actions
are a means for making human services more effective. They
also provide experience in self-government which are
fundamental to democratic citizenship.

All three forms of coproduction are especially important
for human services. These are services which require for
their success the transformation of the behavior of the person
being served. By overlooking coproduction, the public has
been misled into an overreliance on service agents and
bureaucratic organization of human service activities.

Coproduction is, of course, only one aspect of citizens'
participation in public policy. Voting, campaigning, demonstrating, testifying, and petitioning influence the choice of
public officials and their choices of laws, rules, budgets, and
other general guidelines for public policy. The people have in
these activities a set of tools for checking the excesses of
public officials, redirecting public goals, and developing their
own citizenship. Coproduction is a necessary complement to
these more familiar kinds of citizens' participation.

NOTES

(1)   Carole Pateman, Participation and Democratic Theory
      (London: Cambridge University Press, 1970).
(2)   Victor R. Fuchs, The Service Economy (New York: Basic
      Books, Inc., 1973), pp. 357-374; and Harvey A. Garn,
      "Human Services on the Assembly Line," Evaluation 1
      (May 1976): 36, 41-42.
(3)   Not everything that teachers or doctors or police officers
      do is "human service" according to this definition. Ex-
      pelling a student, isolating a patient with a contagious
      disease, and arresting a robber are all activities in which
      the subject of the agent's attention is not expected to

benefit. In this sort of action, the agent's primary interest is in protecting others from the danger posed by the person being restrained.

(4) Stephen D. Cupps, "Emerging Problems of Citizen Participation," Public Administration Review 37 (September/October, 1977): 478.

(5) Ibid., p. 485.

(6) Richard L. Cole, Citizen Participation and the Urban Policy Process (Lexington, Mass.: D.C. Heath, 1974), p. 312.

(7) Stanley B. Greenberg, Politics and Poverty: Modernization and Response in Five Poor Neighborhoods, Wiley Series, vol. 5 of Urban Research, ed. Terry N. Clark (New York: John Wiley, 1974), pp. 42-72.

(8) Gabriel Almond and Sidney Verba, The Civic Culture (Boston: Little, Brown, 1965), pp. 168-169.

(9) Ibid., pp. 16-18.

(10) Vincent Ostrom, The Intellectual Crisis in American Public Administration (Tuscaloosa, Ala: University of Alabama Press, 1973), p. 92.

(11) Michael Lipsky, "Street Level Bureaucracy and the Analysis of Urban Reform," in Neighborhood Control in the 1970s, ed. Gorge Frederickson (New York: Chandler, 1973), p. 105.

(12) Ostrom, Intellectual Crisis in Public Administration, pp. 102-113.

(13) These three types of citizen participation in police services delivery are being studied as part of the Police Services Project. Observational and interview data were collected regarding police patrolmen in 60 neighborhoods in the Rochester, New York; St. Louis, Missouri; and Tampa-St. Petersburg, Florida metropolitan areas. The project is funded by the Division of Applied Research of the National Science Foundation. It is directed by Elinor Ostrom and Roger B. Parks at Indiana University in Bloomington and myself at the University of North Carolina at Chapel Hill.

(14) Daniel Katz, Barbara Gutek, Robert L. Kohn and Eugenia Barton, Bureaucratic Encounters (Ann Arbor, Mich.: University of Michigan Press, Institute for Social Research, 1975), p. 180.

(15) Lipsky, "Street Level Bureaucracy and the Analysis of Urban Reform," p. 106.

(16) Herman Goldstein, Policing a Free Society (Cambridge, Mass.: Ballinger, 1977), p. 112

(17) Morton Bard, "The Unique Potentials of the Police in Interpersonal Conflict Management." Paper presented at the Annual Meeting of the American Association for the Advancement of Science; The First National Conference of IOSGT, held in Washington, D.C., December 29, 1972.

(18) Frank Levy, Arnold J. Meltsner, and Aaron Wildavsky, Urban Outcomes: Schools, Streets and Libraries, volume in Oakland Project series (Berkeley: University of California Press, 1974).

(19) Jane Jacobs, The Death and Life of Great American Cities (New York: Random House, 1961).

(20) Hubert G. Locke, "The Evolution of Contemporary Police Service," in Local Government Police Management, ed. Bernard L. Germire (Washington, D.C.: The International City Management Association, 1977), p. 15.

(21) George Washnis, Citizen Involvement in Crime Prevention (Lexington, Mass.: D. C. Heath, 1976).

(22) Harrell R. Rodgers, Jr. and Charles S. Bullock III, Law and Social Change: Civil Rights Laws and Their Consequences (New York: McGraw-Hill, 1972).

(23) Washnis, Citizen Involvement in Crime Prevention, pp. 136-137.

(24) Carl Gersuny and William R. Rosengren, The Service Society (Cambridge, Mass.: Schenkman, 1973), p. 308.

(25) William Ker Muir, Jr., Police: Streetcorner Politicians (Chicago, Ill.: University of Chicago Press, 1977), p. 277.

(26) See ibid., and Ostrom, The Intellectual Crisis in American Public Administration, p. 110.

(27) Robert Rosenthal and Lenore Jacobson, "Pygmalion in the Classroom," in Bureaucracy and the Public eds. Elihu Katz and Brenda Danet (New York: Basic Books, 1973), pp. 375-388.

(28) Jonathan Kozol, Death at an Early Age (Boston: Houghton Mifflin, 1967), p. 121.

(29) See Albert J. Reiss, Jr., Police and the Public (New Haven: Yale University Press, 1971), pp. 29-31; and William Muir, Police: Streetcorner Politicians.

(30) Muir, ibid., pp. 119-120.

(31) Eliot Friedson, "The Impurity of Professional Authority," in Institutions and the Person, eds. Howard S. Becker, Blanche Geer, Davis Reisman and Robert S. Weiss (Chicago: Aldine, 1968), pp. 25-34.

(32) Milton Davis, "Variations in Patients' Compliance with Doctors' Advice: An Empirical Analysis of Patterns of Communications," in Bureaucracy and the Public, eds. Katz and Danet, p. 369.

(33) Ibid.

(34) Norval Morris, The Future of Imprisonment (Chicago, University of Chicago Press, 1974).

(35) Morris's suggestions are now being tried experimentally by the U.S. Bureau of Prisons at the Butner Federal Correctional Facility in North Carolina.

(36) Reiss, Police and the Public, p. 220.

12 The Foundations of Political Participation
Prodosh Aich

The western parliamentary democracies have discovered citizens
at the local level. Members of the communities are dissatisfied
with the amount of opportunity for participation, and
government and political parties are anxious about the issue.
Their dilemma is obvious: Should members of communities
participate in decision making in government and enterprise to
a greater extent? How would the entrepreneurs react? Is
decreasing economic growth the price of extended
participation? Can the increasing annoyance, disinterest, and
weariness of the citizen with state affairs receive adequate
attention without creating disinterest among the entrepreneurs?
How can unemployment be justified when private enterprises
show increasing profits?

Politicians, administrators, and scientists notice these
issues and occasionally identify them as problems and
temporary crises, but seldom as social contradictions. Since
there seems to be too little time for analysis, organized social
groups turn rashly to crisis management. Quite understandably, anxiety predominates. What value has parliamentary democracy if citizens cannot participate even at the local
level? Thus, we read in a popular commentary on Gemeindeordnung (rules in the community) in the Federal Republic of
Germany:

> The public affairs at the level of local government
> are still substantially transparent for the individual
> citizen. He has personal interest in them, feels that
> the affairs concern him directly and therefore is
> most easily ready to participate in active "politics."
> In this way the local Selbstverwaltung [self
> government] becomes, just to use the often quoted
> word, a "school of democracy," in the positive sense

of the word. The liveliness of democracy comes from
this interest and willingness for participation of the
citizens in public affairs. The opportunity for
public activities, a chance to share responsibility in
the local government, awakens and increases interest
in more widespread, less-transparent affairs of the
State and of the Federation. This opens up the way
for the citizens to the State, opens their view to
political reality, and makes them responsible bearers
of political reshaping. If there is no opportunity for
citizens to reshape political affairs, then it is quite
difficult for them to find their way to the State.(1)

   Participation by all citizens in the community is the
prerequisite of Selbstverwaltung. Philosophers, social
scientists, and legal scholars agree that without democratic
practice at the level of Gemeinde there can never be a
democratic state. The main objective in a democratic society
should, therefore, be to assure that all persons, at least as
far as possible, can participate in self-government. Many
programs, models, and theories exist to bring this about, but
social scientists tend to move skillfully around the real
problem, the real issue of participation. Since the
prerequisites for participation are distributed unequally, the
supposed "nonparticipation" of the majority is not entirely
accidental. The duty of social scientists and philosophers
should be to describe as precisely as possible the
circumstances under which the quality of participation becomes
so unequal and not to waste time with reflections, so-called
theory, and intellectual stunts that present merely the
appearance of extensive participation.
   The physical and social changes in a community are the
result of specific planning activities such as city development,
slum clearance, reconstruction of old localities, traffic
planning, and industrial planning; they are also the result of
a comprehensive approach to planning by regional, state, and
federal authorities. However, despite the appearance that
there is local involvement, this multiplicity of planning
activities does not reflect a demand for such change by the
inhabitants that are affected. Rather, most changes are the
result of settlement programs for economic reasons that are
planned nationally and implemented on various levels at the
direction of the federal government. The goal of such
planning is to accelerate the movement of goods and of human
beings from one place to another. Referred to as "mobility" in
sophisticated, academic terms, this movement continues to be,
thanks to social scientists, the symbol of progress in a diligent
democratic nation.
   The local citizens carry the burdens of the settlement
programs. One of these burdens is unemployment. Although

the planners maintain that new jobs can be created only if high profits spark new investment, their use of the remarkable term Strukturelle Arbeitslosigkeit (joblessness caused by structural changes) conceals that unemployment is a consequence of their programs which require new investment capital. The other dubious rewards of the programs for local citizens include traffic jams, the elimination of reasonable rents, land speculation, and pollution. The original inhabitants are often forced to leave as the town is transformed into shopping centers and supermarkets with exorbitant prices.

Although the local governments continue to sanction the planning decisions of the higher levels of government and can theoretically oppose them under the right of Selbstverwaltung in the constitution, the communities have in fact little opportunity to act otherwise. The average citizen is faced with the results of the decision-making process and has no chance to become involved in or even to observe that process. Yet the entire procedure is part of the accepted legal framework. Given this state of affairs, how is it possible for a citizen to influence the decision-making process?

Consider the situation within the local political unit. The fundamental idea of Selbstverwaltung is embodied in the election of delegates by citizens to represent their interests in a parliamentary body. Because the elected officials cannot perform administrative duties in addition to fulfilling their responsibilities for overseeing the interests of the citizens, the local government recruits administrative personnel to conduct the actual business of Selbstverwaltung. The duty of the elected body is to ensure that these personnel carry out its decisons accordingly.

However, in practice, the community is separated from the decision-making process by political parties. The relationship between the citizens and their representatives is not direct, but is rather mediated by political parties in ways that neglect local interests. Political parties develop their programs at a central level, not at the local level, which means that the party nominees take positions determined less by the concrete needs of the local inhabitants than by the elements of the party program. In addition, the inclination of the nominees is not toward local interests, for the choice of nominees reflects the power constellations within the party rather than the qualifications of nominees to deal with local interests. Local self-government is seen by nominees as merely a stepping stone to careers at the national level. The temporary stay of such party nominees at the local level has serious disadvantages for the local people. Whenever there is a conflict between local and national interests the councillors who have national ambitions choose the alternative favorable to the national interest if they are confident that the public will not learn of their decisions. Unfortunately, there are ample opportunities for the councillors to conceal such machinations from the public.

As a result of both the mechanisms within political parties and the necessity of administrative personnel, the specialists at the local level are administrative rather than elected specialists. They are consultants who do not have the right of decision. However, because they control the information process, the administrative specialists actually determine the decisions that are made by the honorary councillors. The councillors are dependent on the administrative specialists for essential information and well-balanced assessments of proposals because of their superior knowledge and because the councillors are not in a position to receive and process such information. The decisions of the bureaucracy provide the basis for the decisions of the special committees and then the municipal council. This process occurs in private, since important committee meetings are not open to the public. Although their reasons differ, both the council and the administration do not want the public to know about the mechanics of the decision-making process. Thus, the real process of decision, even at the local level, is exactly the opposite of what a parliamentary democracy is committed to provide.

The administration in a community is largely independent of the council and provides continuity in political matters as the elected representatives change. The administration is not directly controlled by the council, but is rather placed under an elected administrator, the Gemeindedirektor (Director of the community). This administrator is not elected directly, and is generally a party nominee; he becomes independent of the politics of the council and the party upon election. He has obligations to only the Gemeindeordnung (Community Acts), which are passed by the states. As administrator of the community, it is also his duty to represent local interests against those of higher levels and to further national unity. The relative permanence of the administration, which establishes political stability, ensures its great independence from the changing council. In contrast to the councillors, who are elected for four or five years, the Director and heads of the departments within the administration are elected for a significantly longer period, usually twelve years. By the end of their terms alone, the administrators gain authority and power over both the citizens and the councillors.

The local administration is subject to the influence of the other nonelected administrations on the state and national levels, but these relationships ultimately reinforce the autonomy of the local administration with regard to the citizens and the council. A subadministration of the state, the Mittelinstanz, oversees that the Selbstverwaltung is

administered within the laws.   Also the state and national
administrations directly influence the local administration and
ensure its efficient and unified operation through bodies
referred to as Ubertragener Wirkungskreis (regional
authorities).   These administrations create even more distance
between the local administration and the council and citizens.
The citizen, who pays the costs of these various administrations, is unaware of the influences that the higher ones have
on the local one.   However, the mediating position of the local
administration between the council and the higher level
administration increases its authority and power.   Directly
linked to the higher levels, the local administration has the
power to withhold information concerning the higher levels
from the councillors, who are, again, completely dependent
on the local administration's services.

The consequence of this process is that the elected representatives of the citizens are joined in the decision making
process by the administration.   In order to maximize his
political profile, a councillor will establish a personal working
relationship with administrators who will provide resources,
such as information, that might otherwise be inaccessible.
The extent of close relationships varies from councillor to
councillor, but they are essential because of the authority of
the administration and the power of the administrator.   It
seems to be absolutely impossible to establish democratic
mechanisms to supervise the activities of the administration
and to exercise control over its information resources.

Yet even the administration does not possess unlimited
power, for it is restriced by social and economic conditions.
Its monopoly of information and control of decisions is limited
to certain areas.   Also, powerful citizens, whose decisions
have indirect and direct consequences for the income of the
community, influence the decisions of the administration and
compete for control of information.

The administration is able to control the activities of the
council only if the council is convinced of the efficiency of the
administration.   However, efficiency is a relative term and not
without its contradictory aspects. The administration is blamed
for a decline in the income of the community and for overt
discontent.   As a result, the strategy of the administration is
to prove its efficiency and effectiveness by providing income
growth figures and satisfying influential citizens, thereby
eliminating complaints, which disturb the apparent general
satisfaction of the citizens. Although it does not necessarily
have informal consultations with the powerful citizens of the
community, the administration processes important decisions in
such a way that its authority and power cannot be challenged
by the council, which is in itself powerless.   But the
administration frequently makes contacts with such citizens and
negotiates with them to learn the limits for compromise.   The

strategy is to preserve the authority of the administration publicly and to make the necessary concessions to the powerful citizens privately. Such arrangements are routine.

There is a wide gap between the kind of governance that the democratic rights of citizens entitle them to and the kind of governance they are actually being subjected to. The less powerful have recognized that their party representatives do not represent their interests. However, they also realize that they are faced with limited alternatives in voting because other parties and their nominees seem no better. As a result, their discontent is expressed in either resignation or protest.

It is not evident to the majority of citizens, though, how the interests of the powerful minorities are served. On the surface, the rules of the political game are scrupulously followed. The council and administration have developed a counterstrategy to camouflage the disadvantages for the majority of decisions that favor special interests: They argue that the developments were inevitable and maintain goodwill, and point out that things could be worse. In the long run, however, it is impossible to conceal that many decisions result from the influence of certain interests.

It is obvious that the dissatisfaction of the majority is irreversibly increasing as they realize that these so-called inevitabilities are always disadvantageous for them. The contradiction between the democratic commitment to equality and the actual existence of permanent, unequal distributions is becoming apparent even to them. One consequence of this development has been the emergence of action groups which attempt to challenge decisions in which the disadvantages are obvious. These groups generally have little success.

The relationship of the council and the administration is characterized by a fundamental contradiction that many administrative experts have long recognized. Because so-called self-government is dependent on the interests of powerful citizens, its actions must focus on those interests which leads inevitably to disadvantages for the vast majority of the community. This contradiction is identifiable at all levels. At the national level in the Federal Republic of Germany, the socialist-liberal coalition government frankly confesses that the government must depend on private capital investment to decrease unemployment. And the willingness of private capital owners to invest depends, in turn, on the expectations for profit maximization in the prevailing market, not on any considerations of social policy or morality.

Confronted by this general and unresolvable contradiction, elected bodies and administrations alike at all levels are forced to devise a number of explanations and to promise a series of social-political solutions. It is nearly inevitable, therefore, that the offer of political participation is put forward. It is not all coincidental that the

Stadtebauforderungsgesetz (City Reconstruction Act) of the Federal Republic passed as late as 1971 and the Bundesbaugesetz (Federal Housing Law) passed in 1977 included provisions for some sort of participation. Experts recognize that the offer of participation is limited to hearings only and that those who have to be heard must be directly affected by planned activities. Ultimately the decision of who is allowed to be involved lies with the administrative authority, which offers the hearing.

This type of participation has two advantages for the planning administration. The first is that it can avoid certain mistakes. The second is that the administration has sufficient time to invent strategies of camouflage to console the citizens and to emphasize the priority of general over individual interests. If the administration fails to console the citizens, then protest actions generally follow. In this way, the activities of so-called action groups and the offer of participation develop from the same source, which is the above-mentioned contradiction.

Because of the traditional inequitable distribution of goods, a small number of citizens have always been more influential than others in the decision-making process. The active citizens are listened to by the ruling group to an extent. But there is no doubt that these citizens are supplied with misinformation, rationalizations, and various appeals by the ruling groups. But now, discussions of action groups and of models of participation take place in public; it is puzzling that the discussions are not still held privately which would prevent numerous problems.

Two contradictory explanations are offered by social scientists. They agree that the quality of interpersonal relations has become highly complex as a result of industrial development, which is characterized by vast differentiation of divisions of labor. From this common basis, the analyses diverge. The first position is that citizens cannot exercise adequate control over society because of their personal responsibilities and the complexities of society. They should elect leaders they feel are confident to run the complex social machinery with the assistance of impartial technicians. Confidence in representatives is seen to be better than the exercise of defective and insufficient control. The second position is that citizens must learn to articulate their interests and to promote them through social conflict in order to overcome their helplessness vis-a-vis the administration and elected bodies. Otherwise, the democratic society will fail because the citizens would become totally resigned and would withdraw. Moreover, the social and political decisions of our age have such far-reaching consequences that they should not be left to a few specialists. Social reality seems to support the second position; there are widespread cries about the

necessity of active participation for the achievement of real
democracy.

However, although the conclusions of the two positions
are contradictory on the surface, they can be reconciled to an
extent. First, they both describe the prevailing social
practice. Second, while public discussion emphasizes the
second position, social and political actions are directed by the
realities of the first position. The administrations and elected
bodies recognize that the decision-making processes are more
efficient without citizen participation, but realize that the
absence of participation could have unpleasant consequences
for them. They use apparent participation as a placebo to
forestall rebellion by the underprivileged majority. It might
even be cynically suggested that members of local government
would never talk about participation and action groups if there
were sufficient guarantees based on scientific investigation that
the discriminated majority would not become disgruntled.
However, social scientists are unable to predict precisely the
actions and reactions of citizens. This is because the
acquisition of knowledge and skills demanded of the
underprivileged by the industrial job market produces an
inherent desire for emancipation.

Recognition of this desire for emancipation stands behind
certain offers of more participation and different models of
participation in various areas, regardless of the amount of
sincerity and earnestness of those demanding them. The
demands are used by many as camouflage to make a show of
goodwill toward the majority and to indicate the "objective"
difficulties of exercising that goodwill in actual practice. The
question arises whether the demands and offers for
participation lead to and, indeed, must lead to exactly the
opposite of increased democracy.

A number of programs, models, and theories have been
developed to bring about public participation. The degree of
participation varies among groups because of the inequities in
the distribution of prerequisites for participation. In addition,
the contemporary offers of and demands for public
participation involve the ancient technique of exercising power,
"divide and rule."(2)

The main point is that powerful groups have to win over
certain others to secure their positions, and participation helps
these groups consolidate their power. The recruitment of only
part of the members of society weakens the force of the public
will. Because of the inequality of opportunities for
participation, the extension of more intensive participation
will reinforce inequality, thus contradicting the goal of the
demand. The social reality will be distorted, and the majority
will be blamed for lack of participation.

There are several obvious prerequisites to political
participation in society, in which the hierarchy is determined

by achievements. Those who actively participate in a parliamentary democracy are better educated and have higher incomes. These are the social characteristics of the local councillors. Such citizens have the requisite skills for the exercise of power and are more useful to those who are in a position to offer participation to others. The rest of the population, the vast majority, is excluded from participation in two ways. First, information is hoarded. Second, the majority is kept from developing skills to process information effectively. If information does leak out, the inability of the majority to use it ensures that they will not be able to participate.

Although social scientists are not legitimized to advance the demand for increased participation on behalf of the nonparticipants, they have a duty to demand the establishment of the prerequisites for participation guaranteed in the constitution. The crucial prerequisite is the flow of information. It is more than a scandal that social scientists are not concerned with the fact that certain information is not available for research because it is withheld by the administration for bargaining purposes.

This demand in itself will not lead to extended participation, but a more exact description of the factors limiting equality of participation by the nonparticipants - not the demand for more participation by traditionally powerful groups - will finally arise.

NOTES

(1)   Luersen/Neuffer et al., Kommentar zur Gemeindeordnung, 1973, S.57. Translation by the author.

(2)   Prodosh Aich (ed.), Wie demokratisch ist Kommunal-politik? Gottingen: Schwartz Verlag, 1977. See my introduction.

13 Participation and Local Politics in Marxist Theory and Practice

Adalbert Evers and Juan Rodrigues-Lores

Foreign influences, especially Anglo-American ones, have dominated German discussion of participation and local politics during the postwar era. Elitist and pluralist theorization, advocacy planning, and implementation research are factors in the German debate. In contrast to the tradition in terms of which this debate is carried on, Marxist analysis regards political participation as inseparable from the formation of social classes and class structures. It examines participation in terms of the state's relation to antagonistic economic classes and the parties, unions, and other institutions they create. Similarly, it views local politics not merely as an extension of those of the national state, but rather as a potentially independent arena for strategic class opposition or, to use Gramsci's terms, for the attainment of hegemony by the working class.

Despite their German origins, Marxist concepts of democracy and the state have become increasingly unfamiliar in the Federal Republic.

GERMAN SOCIALISM AND LOCAL POLITICS

At the turn of the century, the German Social Democrats, like the ideological avant garde of capitalism,(1) attempted to reconcile capital and the working class. Kautsky's centrism, for example, sought to bridge the gap between the representatives of bourgeois democracy on the one hand and the working class on the other. Kautsky's theories played an important role in the controversies surrounding a general strike.

Later, perceiving the survival capacities of monopoly capitalism, Social Democratic revisionists discarded the theory that the collapse of that system was imminent. In so doing, they renounced revolutionary tactics and implicitly accepted the ideology of capitalistic rationalization.(2) This neutralization of capitalistic production relationships was accompanied by a corresponding neutralization of the state. No longer the instrument of inevitable oppression by a single class, the democratic state became a locus of participation in which the proletariat could achieve its own reformist goals. Economic and political reorganization accordingly became a morally neutral problem of pragmatic regulation, a development which is reflected in the creation of the terms "rationalization," "administrative reform," "parliamentary reform", etc. Socialism receded to distant, cloudy horizons as an ethical option toward which the reorganized economy should gradually move through parliamentary reform. For the present, working class organizations were to assist this reform through their economic and political collaboration in the progressive planning and rationalization of capital.

Revisionism also affected pre-World War I Social Democratic attitudes toward local politics. Programs such as those of the SPD Munich convention in 1902 and the Prussian SPD in 1910 attributed a class character to local institutions, regarding them as subsidiary management bodies of the civil state. The latter program asserted the need for social revolution: "Only through the overthrow of class rule can the democratic organization of the municipality be completed and thereby become free for a managerial function which equally promotes the prosperity of all."(3) Yet in practice the municipality represented an arena of political, rather than more far-reaching substructural change. Municipal socialism was no longer a program to break bourgeois hegemony in society and production, but was rather a more limited attempt to promote the workers' welfare within existing political and legal institutions.

The German Social Democrats aimed at an internal democratization of the municipality. New municipal characters were meant to ensure decentralization and self-management on the one hand and voting rights on the other. Such changes did not, however, extend to the economic sphere. The introduction of universal suffrage was the logical culmination of these changes. The SPD's municipal socialism underwent no second phase, and the hope of an autonomous economic base for the municipality remained unfulfilled.

German communists considered the state an instrument of class oppression less ambiguously than did the SPD. Unlike their Social Democratic adversaries, communist theoreticians called not for gradual parliamentary reform, but for the outright elimination of the bourgeois state. They proposed that its place be taken by a proletarian state founded on the direct democracy of workers' soviets. These representative councils in the economic sector were to constitute the primary offensive weapon in the revolution, while a workers' party in the bourgeois parliament would constitute only a preliminary defensive instrument for agitation and propaganda. As Lukacs wrote in 1920, "Wherever a workers' soviet (even in modest forms) is possible, parliamentarianism is superfluous."(4)

This simplified concept of the state as an instrument of class oppression led to confrontation between communists and Social Democrats. Even in the 1970s, every attempt to formulate the problem of political participation is bound to fail as long as differing assessments of the prospects for parliamentary change remain irreconcilable. Similarly, a renewed discussion of democracy at the "base" (autogestion, self-management) cannot escape coming to a theoretical dead end unless it develops an adequate conception of the state. Perhaps, however, ideological and practical developments in Italy and France can point the way out of this theoretical dilemma.

THEORY AND PRACTICE IN ITALY AND FRANCE

Theoretical discussions of the state in Italy and France have been greatly influenced by the thought of Gramsci. His theory of state and democracy sought to reconstitute the dialectical interplay between economy and politics, society and state, the masses and political institutions - relationships that are lost in interpretations that view the state solely as an instrument of class oppression. The recovery of this dialectic provides both a strategy for the transition to socialism and a structural principle for socialism after the transition. The central concept in Gramsci's theory is that of hegemony.

When used to describe the relationship between social classes, hegemony refers to the rule (dominio) of one class over another as well as the intellectual and moral leadership (direzione) of one class over the entire society. For Gramsci, hegemony could be realized in varying forms. The French Revolution established a party hegemony in the Jacobin dictatorship, while modern western societies experience the hegemony of capital within representative democracies. In both cases, centralized state bureaucracy shows an inherent tendency to "deny the contradictory forces at the basis of society" and to promote a "lack of initiative from the mass of the people."(5)

Gramsci argued that the way to socialism in the developed capitalist nations lay not in the utilization of the bourgeois state for socialistic goals, but rather in the creation of proletarian hegemony in social and industrial relationships. Before conquering the state, the proletariat must dominate society. It must assume moral and intellectual leadership. Hegemony, he said, can be achieved through an anticapitalist "historical bloc" that includes the agricultural and intellectual classes. The formation of this revolutionary coalition requires, however, a "moral and intellectual reform of the masses" and new fundamental institutions to replace their bourgeois counterparts.

Rejecting traditional ideological categories, Gramsci's theory envisages a dynamic social group which leads society and claims hegemony as the basis of political rule. The "new type of state" therefore means a new concept of power, a new state form realized from below, from the base institutions of hegemony in economy and society. Gramsci's democratic program reverses the conventional participation debate: political participation of the masses presupposes their own social, cultural, and economic power as well as a transformed and revitalized theory of the state.

Social and economic changes in the West since the late 1960s have stimulated a lively debate over participation. Numerous societal institutions such as the factory, the school, the city, and the family have fallen into crisis and encountered increasing antiauthoritarianism and insubordination. People have politicized these institutions in the attempt to gain greater control over their own destinies and to overcome the dichotomy between private and public spheres.

These changes have prompted the creation of institutions at the base of society which challenge the accepted, restricted definitions of politics and the state. Such institutions, spawned particularly by the urban movements in Italy and parts of France, create a potential for working-class hegemony in Gramsci's sense. Rejecting both Soviet and Social Democratic theory and practice, they provide the prerequisites for the transfer of state power to the base of society even before the transition to socialism.

The urban movement gave the impetus for a new definition of participation and local politics. In Italy, the movement arose from the failure of the center-left government's reforms and the struggles in the factories and universities during the "hot autumn" of 1969. Urban protest grew primarily where living conditions were worst, in ghettos inhabited by recent arrivals from southern Italy who had not yet found jobs. These people simply lacked housing and money to pay rent. Thus 20,000 dwellings were illegally occupied in Rome between 1969 and 1972, and, in Milan, approximately 10,000 were occupied illegally in 1970 alone. Thirty-five thousand families took part in a rent strike in 1972. These spreading protests gave birth to demands for rent control and expanded public housing.

Very soon, these urban protest movements underwent a qualitative change. The growing Italian economic crisis - unemployment, inflation, and decline in real income - broadened the social base of urban protest beyond the groups on the margin of society. The large working-class political organizations and the unions were forced to concern themselves with urban distress. Within a few years, the movement assumed relative stability through the formation of district councils and renters' unions, analogous to the workers' councils in the spheres of production.

Urban struggle in France has been much less intense than in Italy, with the possible exception of the area around Paris. There, urban discontent reflects resistance to various forms of sociospatial segregation: misdirected traffic and urban renewal policies, lack of social services in newly built districts bordering the city, increased costs for rent and public transportation, and deplorable living conditions for Paris's foreign workers. In many cases, urban initiatives there exhibit an interclass character, skilled workers cooperating with small business operators and employees. As flight from the inner city has become increasingly difficult, the middle class has come to support and even dominate some protest initiatives.

In contrast to the Italian situation, no coherent urban movement grew out of the numerous diverse struggles in France. Citizens' protest challenged the logic of capitalistic development, but it did not achieve major qualitative change. Initiatives remained heterogeneous and dispersed. Not directly tied to workers' struggles in the factory, they received only perfunctory recognition from the labor unions. Finally, they failed to create permanent institutions comparable to the Italian district councils and renters' unions.

Despite these differences, the French and Italian urban initiatives share at least one common negative characteristic. In neither country are these initiatives true participatory movements that provide a greater voice for citizens in municipal administration. Rather, they are autonomous social subjects that gradually develop into independent collective groups. Their success or failure depends primarily on the specific national and local context, particularly the reaction of labor unions and parties of the left.

The initial reactions of the established leftist parties must be understood in light of their long practical experience at the local level. The municipal policy of the French and Italian communist parties from before World War II through the late 1960s may be summarized in the phrase "good government." Neither of these parties viewed local control of social services as a step toward "municipal socialism" or believed in the possibility of creating "socialist islands" under a centralized system of government. Consequently, the problem of national politics was duplicated at the local level: on the one hand, there were modest social reforms within the system; on the other, there was utilization of institutional positions for socialist and communist propaganda.

Still largely bound to this traditional program, the established parties tend to exploit the new urban movement for their own parliamentary gains.   Growing dissatisfaction, they calculate, can be translated into a greater number of leftist votes.   At the same time, the existing parties attempt to integrate and slow down the new urban movement in the name of an abstract "leadership of the working class."   This attempt is likely to fail, however, since the urban movements exhibit a radical democratic impulse which cannot be channeled into subjection by a political party.   Further, the urban protests reflect a deep distrust of bureaucratic reform policies, a distrust which cannot easily be transformed into a vague dissatisfaction expressed solely at the ballot box.   The reaction of the traditional left - effective management and ideological paternalism - does not come to grips with the problems and potential of new urban protest.

The urban movement challenges traditional notions of participation in representative democracies in two ways.   First, it articulates precise social demands which conflict with the logic of capitalist development.   Particularly in Italy it concerns itself primarily not with better management, but with the extension of social services as a means for general redistribution of goods and living space in the city.   Second, it redefines the relationships between parties and social movements and between governmental institutions and organized countervailing powers; in short, it redefines the relationship between the state and genuine democracy.   Leftist parties are forced to recognize the independence of urban movements which, while sharing their modes of organization and their opposition to the bourgeois state, refuse to accept subjection to any external force.   Attempting to win support from the expanding social movement, these parties give to state institutions under their influence or control a new internal structure more closely corresponding to the progressive forces of society.   In this context belong the decentralization demands of the French and Italian left and other efforts to create new governmental and societal forms.

In many Italian leftist-controlled municipalities, new forms of participation are being created at the levels of district councils, open district commissions, and local cooperatives. In addition to these interclass possibilities, new working class councils in the district and the factory can combine with the unions to attain a greater voice in municipal administration.

This effort is less advanced in France, with the exception of that in cities such as Grenoble.   The major parties of the left attempt to organize local and communal opposition, but the centralization of the French state hinders social change at the local level. As in Italy, however, the leftist parties in France are not attempting to create a ready-made alternative power structure, but are trying instead to achieve eventual hegemony through appropriation and transformation of existing state institutions. The French socialist party, for example, has proposed expanded "communal commissions" composed of representatives of municipal and district councils, unions, government administration, and citizens' groups. It has suggested greater popular control over social and cultural services as well as expanded opportunities for local input in open sessions of the district councils.

The differing, if not conflicting, objectives of urban movements and Marxist parties obviously create a certain tension within the left. The two groups engage simultaneously in conflict and cooperation, even communities under leftist control. On the one hand, leftist forces do not wish to create difficulties for their own parties or local governments; on the other hand, they desire to utilize effectively the institutional power they have already attained. Thus, the participation debate cannot remain theoretical and abstract; it must always refer to a specific socioeconomic and political context.

While in France a certain mystification of the social "base movements" has taken place, in Italy the debate has reached a later stage. The question has been raised of which institutions should take precedence in a social and political opposition bloc. Some suggest that the radical urban groups must yield to existing social institutions, while others regard them as nascent elements of a new political will which is to supersede the traditional state. Two further questions are whether the urban movements are not threatened even by leftist-controlled governmental and semigovernmental institutions and whether cooperation with these established forces could not be perverted into social and political control.

Many of these questions concern the problem of what role new state forms, structures, parties, and urban movements should play in replacing the established political powers. One must ask what concrete forms the hegemony of the "historical oppositional bloc" should take. These are controversial issues within the socialist and Eurocommunist movements and the new left. A certain unity is provided, however, by their agreement on the special role played by participation in local politics in achieving fundamental social change.

PARTICIPATION IN THE FEDERAL REPUBLIC OF GERMANY

The discussion of democracy and participation in Germany has assumed a different character during the past several years.

The failure of the "internal reforms" concept and the isolation of the new-left movement of the 1960s from institutionalized representation have put an end to hopes for the gradual realization of greater participation. An implicit all-party coalition has adopted an ideology of "crisis solution" that is characterized by continual technical modernization combined with an increasing marginalization of workers and citizens whose labor is not directly productive. This ideology seeks to hinder active participation by organizing passive consensus, reviving theories of social partnership, and demanding the self-discipline and restraint of certain economic interest groups. It represses social movements whose objectives do not correspond to its own, and under the pretext of "management" it attempts to form a closer union of state and society that results in paternalistic control over the individual.

In this sort of climate, the prescriptions for improved participation of a decade ago are clearly outdated. Yet despite the prevalence of the crisis-solution ideology, there is increasing unrest in both the unions and in segments of the Social Democratic and Free Democratic parties. In addition, numerous (though heterogeneous) social protest organizations and citizens' action organizations have sprung up. Those in the environmental and energy fields have already assumed the character of genuine social movements.

The forces within the political parties that are searching for alternative approaches to sociopolitical participation have not yet begun serious discussion of ways to broaden representative democracy. Tendentious references to "our free democratic basic order" are calculated to hinder serious consideration of more direct democracy. The scattered urban movements and citizens' action groups, on the other hand, while providing no sufficient answers in and of themselves, indicate the existence of a radical democratic consciousness that insists upon a reformulation of the fundamental issues of democracy and participation.

Despite their promising beginnings, the new social movements still lack an offensive democratic strategy organically tied to their own socioeconomic interests. Just as every successful model of social and economic development implies a corresponding theory of political rule, any effective model of democracy must be tied to specific social interests and demands. Here the progressive forces in West Germany have hitherto fallen short: Lacking any common comprehensive political-economic theory, they have been united only in the important but inherently defensive struggle to preserve fundamental liberal rights against a new authoritarianism. They confront the entrenched political powers merely with those powers' own historical ideals. This defense of traditional bourgeois democracy is unable effectively to integrate and implement the demands of Germany's new social protest initiatives.

The West German left thus lacks a comprehensive, offensive concept of participation and democracy organically united with the nation's new social and economic demands. The need for such a concept, however, is felt not only in socialist and communist circles, but also on the liberal and Social Democratic left. Perhaps the urban initiatives in Italy and France can provide valuable lessons for German theory and practice.

NOTES

(1)   F. Nauman, Mitteleuropa (Berlin: G. Fischer-Verlag, 1915). See also W. Rathenau, Die neue Wirtschaft (Berlin: G. Fischer-Verlag, 1918).

(2)   P.   Hirsch,   ed.,   Das Kommunalprogramm der Social-demokratie PreuBens (Berlin: Verlag   Buchhandlung Vorwurts Paul Singer GmbH, 1911).

(3)   O. Bauer, Rationalisierung - Fehrationalisierung (Wien: Verlag der Wiener Volksbuchhandlung, 1931).

(4)   G. Lukacs, "Zur Frage des Parlamentarismus," Kommunismus, No. 6 (Berlin, 1920): 140.

(5)   A. Gramsci, Opere, Quanderni del carcere, vol. 4 (Turin: Edizioni Einaudi, 1966), p. 155.

V
Health Policy

14 Health Policy Implementation and Corporate Participation in West Germany*
Christa Altenstetter

Like other industrial nations, the Federal Republic of Germany is becoming more of a service society.(1)   In 1955 only 19 percent of the working population was employed in the tertiary sector, whereas 29 percent was employed in it in 1975.   In the health sector, developments have been slightly more rapid.   Of 1,000 employed persons in the tertiary sector in 1955, 14.3 were employed in the health field.   By 1975 the number had risen to 25.5 health workers per 1,000 employed persons. Similarly, health workers represented 1.4 percent of the total German labor force in 1955.   By 1975 their proportion had risen   to   2.6   percent,   with   some   health   occupations experiencing   faster   growth   than   others.   In   1976, approximately 1.7 million people were health workers.   In other words, one out of every 15 employed persons was working in the health sector.(2)   During the same period, the Federal Republic has experienced increases in health expenditures that continue to rise.   In 1970, health expenditures amounted to 6.2 percent of the GNP, but in 1978, they were more than 8 percent of it.   Expenditures for hospital care represented approximately 30 percent of health-insurance expenditures in 1978 and 17 percent in 1960.(3)

Recent   political   debate   has   centered   on   the   crisis   in health and the need to develop policy instruments to contain it and to prevent health costs from rising.   Political debates tend to focus on short-term perspectives.   Often the quality of the

*The   author   gratefully   acknowledges   the   support   of   this research by the International Institute of Management (West Berlin) and the generous leave of absence granted her by the City University of New York.

debate and its focus correspond to overall societal concerns, preferences, and values but diverge from the empirical realities of the subject. The diverse transitions that have taken place in the service sector, transitions that are also cost-causing factors, are often ignored. These transitions include the increasing professionalization of all activities associated with the delivery of services, from highly scientific and technological ones to the delivery of home health and nursing care to the administration of health insurance and the management of sophisticated data and information systems built and staffed by policy actors in the health field. Hardly any area is untouched by substantial and costly change. However, attempts at clarifying what the crisis is all about tend to mystify what is cause and what is effect and who is responsible for the present situation.

The health field is in need of rethinking and restructuring, and that is expensive. But different dimensions of cause and effect should be isolated and examined before a decision is made about whether there is an actual crisis or a limited tolerance for the difficulties of governance - difficulties that are greater when funds for an increasing number of complex and interdependent societal problems are more limited than they are under normal circumstances.(4) The present discussion seems to reflect not only the acceptance of the crisis as a fact but also to incorporate the tendency to look for the causes of the crisis in the private sector rather than in the public sector. To do so, however, means overlooking numerous governmental actions that have contributed to the present situation. The health field in the mid-1970s presents a perfect example of a national debate that is narrow and beclouded by values rather than objective and comprehensive. What is more serious is that the debate lacks solid, up-to-date information about the health sector.

HEALTH AND EMPLOYMENT

The public debate seems to ignore the problem of employment in health services, although occasional proposals have been made about absorbing surplus workers. The health sector is both an important employer and a service sector that produces and consumes costly services. Not surprisingly, those who argue for the reduction of the number of beds and the closing of hospitals are usually national political and trade union leaders, business leaders, and leaders of national associations and national semipublic associations. Depending on the nature of health issues, different federal health bureaucracies are involved. Usually the positions they take are not concerned with how program changes may result in job cuts. The consequences of national recommendations are felt by subnational actors and, in particular, by individual health workers. The irony of the constraints imposed by national policy making is obvious. The issues of unemployment and of cost inflation in the health sector are of national concern. But there are different policy-making entities that deal with these two areas; by definition, the policy instruments that treat unemployment problems are not the same as the ones that treat the problem of inflation.

The health-services sector is crucial not only in that it provides care, but also in that it provides much employment. The health sector has made a valuable contribution to the battle against unemployment. A recent study concludes: "If the demand for health services had experienced developments similar to other areas in 1975, the number of unemployed people would have been higher by about 13 percent than it actually was in 1975."(5)

FUNCTIONAL-ASSIGNMENT POLICIES:
THE BASIC FRAMEWORK

The functional, institutional, and territorial division of authority for making and implementing health decisions between the Bund (the federal government) and the Lander (the states) on the one hand, and between governmental sectors and professional and sickness-fund organizations on the other, is a characteristic feature of the German health policy-making system.(6) Many responsibilities that are vital to the development of national health resources are not within the responsibility of the federal government. For example, the Lander control health-manpower development, training, and accrediting, as well as licensing. They also control hospital matters, the Public Health Services, and environmental and community health. Autonomous professional organizations that are quasipublic agencies are responsible for delivering service and for the geographical and functional distribution of physicians and dentists in private practice. These professional organizations operate nationally and in the Land policy-making system. Similarly, quasipublic organizations concerned with the distribution of sickness funds at both national and Land levels are responsible for health insurance matters. The Federal Committee of Physicians/Dentists and Sickness Funds, with counterparts in the Lander, is at the top of a hierarchically organized system of influential nongovernmental health policy-making bodies. The formal structure consists of delegation of authority to quasipublic organizations that are subject to some mechanisms for professional, bureaucratic, and legal accountability. Another formal aspect of the structure is that general authority for passing legislation and for issuing regulations on health insurance and health-care delivery remains with the federal government in some areas and with the Lander in others.

This large and complex web of public, semipublic, and private organizations that implements health policy in the health-services sector is financed not only by public and private health insurance (and some out-of-pocket funds), but also by an array of intergovernmental financing mechanisms. Financing by grants-in-aid is particularly prevalent in the areas of manpower development and training programs, the construction of facilities and hospital planning, the contracting for and the distribution of costly equipment and medical technology, and the Public Health Services. As a result of the dominance of these two modes of health financing, insurance and intergovernmental financing, and of the functional and territorial allocation of decision-making authority in health, numerous interdependencies have developed among governmental bureaucracies and between public bureaucracies and those in semipublic and private organizations. However, the nature and the extent of such linkages, their effects on implementation processes and on the impacts of national decisions, and, finally, the ways in which such interdependencies have changed over time are largely unexplored.

"Health policy" as a whole consists of an accumulation of numerous individual policy statements, decisions, and actions taken at different times. Because they are made and passed by different processes (legislative and administrative processes and, occasionally, court decisions), interdependencies, structures and functions are different in each major policy and program area. In terms of policy areas, there is a difference between policies that address the delivery of medical care in physician's offices and policies that address the delivery of medical care in short-term hospitals. In terms of program aspects, the following functional areas need to be examined: financing, planning and resource allocation, standards of care and service delivery, and, finally, the role of information generation and management in formulating new decisions and in administering activities that depend heavily on information.

Some general findings on the meaning and the objectives of "health policy" are available. For example, decisions and actions taken over time do not always add up to consistent trends in objectives.(7) Increased governmental influence in defining through legislation and regulation the content of health policy within the framework of public health insurance has tended to reduce the decentralized, autonomous decision-making authority of local insurance carriers. On the one hand, these decisions follow a long-standing and time-honored objective, namely to provide as large a segment of the population with fairly comprehensively defined coverage that is mandated nationally. On the other hand, another long-standing and equally important objective, the self-governance of insurance carriers, has been compromised in favor of further bureaucratization. In a way, public health policy making, supported by successive party and coalition governments over the last twenty-five years, has almost made a farce of the concept of self-governance or Selbstver-waltung.(8) That self-governance serves symbolic political functions becomes even more evident because in a period when decisions have been increasingly centralized, political rhetoric has stressed some kind of administration that should be responsive to citizens' needs, or burgernahe Ver-waltung.(9) However, stressing the participation of citizens when no important decisions can be made at low levels of administration is both politically astute and cynical. People alienated from government are receptive to such promises. Truly responsive administration would require that there be real rather than token input into decision making of local demands and needs. The emphasis on responsive administration is also manipulative.

POLICY ANALYSIS, ORGANIZATIONS, AND INHERITANCE

For some time, much of what was subsumed under the heading of policy analysis has revealed not only a strong economic orientation but also a basically nonhistorical orientation in both theoretical formulation and approach. Institutional and interorganizational analyses reveal numerous constraints on the implementation of national health decisions. A new appreciation of historical dimensions of these analyses is emerging because failures to provide innovative decisions can be attributed to many functional and structural processes initiated decades ago.(10) Agreements reached in past decades about how and with whom business should be conducted continue to apply today. Furthermore, the institutional and personal behavior of those participating in such processes is conditioned by historical patterns and styles of governance and conflict resolution.

The importance of the historically conditioned patterns of participation contradicts the assertion made elsewhere that the organizational arrangements of present-day policy issues and instruments may not matter over a long period of time.(11) Although this conclusion is correct for some aspects of implementation, it is incorrect for others. As individual programs and the events that change linkages and elements of implementation are studied, the significance of the heritage of patterns of governance and conflict resolution becomes clear.

THE INSTITUTIONAL CONTEXT: MEDICAL MARKETS
AND MULTI-INSTITUTIONAL SERVICE ARRANGEMENTS

Medical care is consumed in private offices and in hospitals
through the purchase of services in "markets" that are
controlled by full-time bureaucracies representing either
professional and governmental interests or the interests of
sickness funds and hospitals. These bureaucratic
organizations serve as intermediaries between compulsory-
membership organizations and the individual members in the
cases of policies that affect the delivery of medical services
in private practice. Hospital associations based on voluntary
membership serve as intermediaries between individual
hospitals and other policy actors. These intermediaries
negotiate prices, contractual conditions, rewards, and
sanctions that are binding on individual patients who are
members of a sickness fund, on physicians, and on hospital
and individual sickness funds.

In 1977, Germany had 62,057 physicians who were
employed full-time in public and private hospitals and 54,974
physicians who practiced privately. Of a total of 2,297
short-term hospitals, 936 (40 percent) were public hospitals
providing about 54 percent of all beds, 931 (41 percent) were
private nonprofit hopsitals providing 42 percent of all beds,
and the remaining 428 were private, profit-making institutions.
In addition, local or areawide sickness funds in 1975 employed
a total of 38,137 persons (plus an additional 900 people who
worked for the peak associations in the Land organizations or
in their national headquarters).(12) In matters concerning
hospitals or private practices, field offices of the Land
government, county offices, or local governmental agencies
play roles. Whereas personal and institutional providers are
involved primarily in the delivery of medical services, the
remaining agencies are engaged primarily in facilitating and
controlling, in data-collecting services, in certifying service
providers, in bilateral service agreements for fees and hospital
charges, and in multilateral and multicentered hospital planning
processes.

These producers, service administrators, hospitals, and
sickness funds are integral parts of loosely structured interorganizational systems of relationships that provide services
not only to 90 percent of the population that is covered by
public health insurance but also to approximately 10 percent of
the population that has private insurance and to private
payers of medical bills.

TABLE 14.1. DOMINANT INTERMEDIARY ACTORS IN NEGOTIATING AND DECISION-MAKING SYSTEMS IN THE AMBULATORY AND HOSPITAL CARE SECTORS

Type of Care Sector	Negotiating and Decision-Making Area	Governmental Actors				Professional			Nongovernmental Actors — Insurance Carriers			Nongovernmental Actors — Hospital Interests		
		Federal	Land	Areawide	Local	Federal	Land	Doctor	Federal	Land	Fund	Federal	Land	Hospital
Medical Care	– fee for service	L+SR	SR			AND	AND	AND	AND	AND				
	– planning	L+SR	SR			AND	AND		AND	AND				
	– professional standards of service delivery	L+SR	L+SR			AND	AND	AND		AND				
	– information systems and management	L+SR	SR				AND		AND					
Hospital Care and Hospital Resources	– financing of hospital resources	L+AND+F	L+AND+F	OM	AM+F				CA	CA		CA	CA	CA
	– planning of hospital resources	L+SR	L+AND	CA	CA			CA		CA		CA	CA	
	– professional standards of hospital care	L+SR	L+SR	SR+OM			AND		CA			CA		
	– hospital charges	L+AND+CA	SR	SR+OM							AND+OM	CA		AND+OM OM
	– information systems and management	SR+AND	SR+AND	SR+OM	OM						OM		AND+OM	OM

Key

L	Legislative Role
AND	Administrative Negotiating and Decision-Making Role
CA	Consultative/Advisory Role
SR	Supervisory and Regulatory Role
OM	Operations and Management
F	Financing Role

Hierarchical, Multilayered, and Exclusive
Interorganizational Negotiating Systems

Depending on the service area, different institutional intermediaries dominate the administrative, negotiating, and decision-making systems. Table 14.1 summarizes the dominant formal actors and the dominant roles that they play in policy matters pertaining to private and hospital medicine and to planning for hospital resources. Dominance is a concept that needs further refinement, but the meaning that suffices for present purposes refers to the existence of major policy actors who exercise legitimate authority in certain functional areas. This dominance has various roots, ranging from historical legitimacy and institution building to official assignment and delegation to the autonomy of a policy sector that has resisted legislative interventions.

Health Care Delivery under Public Health
Insurance: The Streamlining Function of
Organization Structure

Despite the appearance of increased politization and the opening up of health decision making to a larger group of actors, implementation of policy in health affairs is not a process open to many participants. Furthermore, government by advisory committees and government by commission reinforce the closed nature of policy-making circles in governmental as well as in nongovernmental administrative processes, particularly in the gray zone of public and quasipublic interaction.

In the private medical sector, two groups of intermediaries implement practically all aspects of health delivery under public health insurance for 90 percent of the eligible population.(13) The institutional decision makers are health-insurance organizations and the organization of sickness-fund physicians. They are "Korperschaften des offentlichen Rechts" (corporate organizations with public law status). Although this legal designation is not limited to health insurance and physicians' organizations, it is unique in comparison to the rest of German administration and to similar structures abroad. A Korperschaft des offentlichen Rechts has authority to make binding decisions in those matters that are explicitly delegated to it. This legal designation not only conveys considerable authority, but it also serves the function of automatically ascribing to them almost any health matter, to the exclusion of other public or private organizations. Although these two kinds of organizations are on opposite ends of a continuum of interests and goals, each organization defends this legal construction fiercely. Not surprisingly, the blurred lines between the public and private sectors and their respective responsibilities remain. Furthermore, this formal designation camouflages another problem in that the principle of full-fledged bargaining, accepted by the political community at large, would require that there be mechanisms for developing a mix of different kinds of accountability; present procedures, however, tend to stress only the use of selective kinds of accountability the legitimacy of which is rooted, in many instances, in historical circumstances that are quite different from those of the 1970s.

The 100-year history of the relationship between sickness funds and providers and the history of their respective relations with four political regimes have been full of conflict and confrontation as well as alliances. What counts today, however, are the existing legal decision-making structures that have given them strategic positions in health and that reinforce their claims as though they had proprietary rights over health issues.(14)

How strategic this position is can be easily revealed. The scope of matters falling within their authority has increased steadily and includes today practically the whole range of health matters outside of those pertaining to hospitals. Although the governmental sector has increasingly defined health matters through laws and regulations, details of what their content should be are delegated to the policy actors in those intermediary organizations. Thus, despite governmental centralization, government by delegation continues to be important in defining content in the areas of: curative and reparative medicine (diagnostic, therapeutic, rehabilitative); dental care; cancer screening and detection programs; maternal, prenatal, and posnatal care; the provision of health services to anybody in need; dental and medical appliances, fittings, and prescriptions; control medicine for sickness funds and other social insurance programs; industrial medicine; and family planning, sterilization, and abortion.

The main legal, contractual, and organizational linkages between the hierarchically organized system of the sickness funds and the equally hierarchically organized system of physicians' organizations are described below. With few exceptions, these linkages apply to all health areas in the domain of subnational organizations.

Autonomous or quasipublic federal organizations of physicians and sickness funds lay down general binding rules agreed on and issued by the all-powerful Federal Committee of Physicians and Sickness Funds. Collective contractual arrangements have the force of law, are binding on the respective membership organizations, and cannot be changed unilaterally. There are bipartisan committees that regulate licensing and the dispensation of services, that audit claims, and that arbitrate matters between the two opponents in case of disagreement.

By law, physicians' organizations are delegated the responsibility of providing services according to agreements that govern the delivery of health services under health insurance.

The collective decision-making system resembles the federal structure of the political system. For this reason, three organizational layers of the policy-making system can be distinguished. At each level a separate but internally consistent contract is negotiated. The organizational layers of the policy-making system are the federal, Land (state), and local levels. Local contracts constituted exceptions rather than the rule and were given up some time before the July 1977, legislation on cost containment institutionalized and ratified this practice. Now contracts are negotiated at the federal and state levels only.

The federal organizations of sickness funds and physicians are the only contractual partners at the federal level that are engaged in reaching general policy decisions and recommendations. Details connected with licensing, auditing, reimbursement, and arbitration are negotiated and implemented at the state level. De jure, providers and sickness funds are equal partners. De facto, providers have been senior partners. Because of the constraints of limited funds and the political emphasis on the importance of the attitudes of clients, however symbolic it may be, sickness funds are changing from agencies that simply administer public health insurance into agencies that are meant to become involved more significantly in developing and shaping health policies. As this transitional period progresses, the intermediary Land organizations have become more important both in external relations and in relations with their individual local members.

The Present Agenda for Negotiating Systems
in Private Medicine: Geographic Resource
Allocation and the Law on Cost Containment of 1977

In addition to the policy issues, two recent health decisions of the Bundestag set the agenda of these intermediary organizations for interorganizational exchanges, particularly at the Land level. The implementation of the law on cost containment in July 1977, and the law on resources allocation and planning of late 1976 are two major agenda-setting events for the activity of subnational organizations.

Concern over growing imbalances in the distribution of medical and dental manpower was expressed inside and outside the Bundestag in 1970. Legislative policy formation for the solution of geographic imbalances in the provision of medical and dental services has taken several years to be implemented. Plans covering health service needs were expected to be

available by June 1978. By early 1979, no plan was published
in any of the German Lander. Between 1970 and 1979,
however, a change of circumstances occurred in private
medicine. Forecasts about medical manpower made during that
period projected that Germany would suffer from an
undersupply. These forecasts - some made as late as 1975 -
have proved wrong, for the most part. In fact, the present
problem is how to deal with the oversupply of physicians
expected in the early 1980s. Regional disparities in resources
and functional imbalances in specialized services may be solved
automatically, without any kind of intervention and planning.

In the initial phase of preparing the planning guidelines
(1976-1977), the profession developed an information monopoly,
which caused a negative reaction by the sickness funds.
However, in ongoing subnational processes, sickness funds
have prepared themselves very well. Final plans will
eventually reveal whose concepts and objectives will be
adopted. From the very start, it was clear that conflicts
would arise over the territorial scope of planning areas, and
such conflicts have indeed arisen. As a matter of principle,
Land associations of sickness funds have tended to insist on
drawing small planning areas, whereas individual funds have
been more pragmatic. In contrast, professional associations
and individual physicians favor larger planning areas.

A strategy of consensus formation and of conflict
avoidance was chosen for complex interorganizational processes
through which services planning has proceeded. Drastic
departures from the status quo by the German health-care
system should not be expected. However, to the degree that
decision making on issues on which national actors could not or
would not agree is delegated to the subnational arena, some
variations can be expected because of the diversity of
political, social, and health-needs environments in which
planning is carried out.

Planning for health services in the private sector and in
the hospital sector should be coordinated, as political
statements and national programs have repeatedly
recommended. However, such coordination should be
considered a long-term goal because its implementation is
hampered by the existing power structures that dominate each
subsector.

The law on cost containment of July 1977 is an important
milestone in the history of German health policy. A period of
expanding rights and benefits in health services has seemingly
come to an end and is being followed by a period that stresses
financial austerity. Measures taken thus far relate mainly to
providers' income and the prescription of medication. Minor
restrictions on benefits have been imposed. Not all these
measures are new. The most important ones are the following:
An agreed upon rate of increases and/or ceilings on providers'

fees has been applied nationwide; measures to create more cost-consciousness on the part of providers who treat patients and prescribe drugs have been introduced; cost-sharing for medication is being practiced; the legalization of mental out-patient clinics has been accomplished; restrictions on laboratory tests hve been imposed; lists of the contents and the effectiveness of drugs are to be developed; and a national body, Konzertierte Aktion (Concerted Action), is to recommend reform measures, particularly with regard to cost-containment policies.

"Concerted Action" and Private
Medicine and Hospitals

Concerted Action, a national 60-member body composed of a wide spectrum of competing health interests, is to make recommendations through consensus in three main areas: the development of nationwide medical and economic criteria; the rationalization and improvement of effectiveness and efficiency in health-care delivery; and annual rates of increases and/or ceilings on provider reimbursements in the private medical and dental sector, on prescription drugs, and on hospital care. These recommendations are to be made by March 31 of each year on the basis of total health insurance income and annual wage and salary developments. Thus far the Lander, as the dominant governmental actors responsible for hospitals, have argued more successfully than personal providers and pharmacy interests that Concerted Action in health has no authority to make binding recommendations. Such recommendations, say the Lander, violate not only the tenor and individual provisions of the 1972 law, but also the constitutional authority of the Lander in hospital policy and administration. The final answer to the question has not been found. On balance, however, it seems clear that Concerted Action has exerted political pressure. Principal decisions about fees for service were made directly by the federal representatives of private medicine and sickness funds without the advice of Concerted Action.

THE LANDER: GATEKEEPERS OF THE HOSPITAL SYSTEM

Prior to 1969, the Lander were fairly autonomous in hospital matters. In 1969, however, a constitutional amendment transferred responsibility for financing hospital resources to the federal government. The federal government and the Lander have shared financial responsibility for medical schools since 1971 and for short-term general hospitals since 1972.

However, in all matters except financing, the Lander assert their authority.

FINANCING HOSPITAL INVESTMENTS AND
HOSPITAL SERVICES

The 1972 law on hospital financing was a watershed in German hospital policy development and in the short-term hospital sector. It introduced three policy instruments: (a) It required planning for hospital investments, resources, and regional hospital services of high quality in both urban and rural areas; (b) it institutionalized the concept of dual financing of hospitals; and (c) it required the participation of nongovernmental health interests in planning processes.

Since 1972, hospital investment financing(15) has been governed by federal/state intergovernmental financing mechanisms and agreements and by state/local financial arrangements. Federal/state arrangements and the conditions for receiving federal funds are alike for all Lander.(16) However, state/local arrangements vary. Hospitals with more than 100 beds that stood the test of state certificate-of-need programs were included in the hospital-need plans of the Lander and became eligible for reimbursements by public and private health insurance. In theory, operating costs for diagnosis, treatment, care, board, lodging, and wages and salaries were to be covered fully by hospital rates to be paid by sickness funds at the rate agreed on by the individual sickness funds and hospitals. The agreed upon rates are certified by governmental price-setting agencies.

Decentralized Negotiating Systems for
Setting Hospital Charges

In practice, the full coverage of operating costs through hospital charges has not been achieved and practiced everywhere. To implement the federal regulation on user charges, the Lander engaged in various administrative practices. Often what was involved was the adjustment of new goals to routine procedures. In some instances, old practices were changed and adapted to new objectives. It has become obvious that existing negotiating systems, because they are decentralized and involve face-to-face negotiations once a year, have given influence to the main participants, hospitals and sickness funds, that cannot be exercised in the same way by all parties. In this process, sickness funds are not as helpless in facing hospitals as they claim to be. Naturally, what they can do is limited by national law, but whatever opportunity for influence remains, they use successfully.

Because local or county governments are the hospital owners, public hospitals have access to tax funds to cover potential differences between agreed upon service charges and actual operating costs. Private hospitals usually have recourse to neither such funds nor other resources. For this reason, they tend to settle for whatever they can get.

Both individual hospitals and insurance funds are amply assisted by the intermediary Land organizations both in preparing and interpreting cost sheets and comparative analyses of expenditures and in handling strategical and tactical matters at the negotiations themselves. Both sides are represented by multimember delegations. Regional governmental offices have to approve and certify the agreed-upon service charge. In case of disagreement, the network of actors is enlarged to include the central ministry responsible for hospital charges. (This ministry is not the same in all Lander.) When ministry intervention does not produce a result that is acceptable to all parties, the courts decide.

There were inter- and intraregional as well as interhospital variations in the size of daily service charges in the past. Whether these variations can be explained by citing the different sizes, functions, types of ownership, and locations of individual hospitals alone or whether they arose from the varying amounts of political and financial power that pertinent actors exercised is not entirely clear, but there is evidence that indicates that the latter was the case. Furthermore, the form, the significance, and the implementation of "economic monitoring" in hospital negotiations differ from those in the private medical sector.(17) Some would argue that economic monitoring in the hospital sector is nonexistent and, therefore, that economic monitoring has become a prime object for reform.

The definition of what items could be financed by investment funds and their differentiation from those that would be financed through daily charges were controversial issues in 1972 and remain so today. The solution was a political compromise then, and the problem requires a political compromise today. As in the past, insurance carriers are expected to push for a narrow definition of what is to be financed by public insurance, whereas hospitals and state and local governments continue to defend the status quo. Insurance carriers and hospitals continue to favor the present practice of direct negotiations and to oppose any increase in government influence over the setting of hospital service charges. However, state governments intend to acquire more influence in this policy area.

CENTRAL CONTROL OF <u>LAND</u> HOSPITAL
PLANNERS OVER HOSPITAL PLANNING

The 1972 federal legislation required that the <u>Lander</u> develop hospital-need plans, multiyear programs, and annual construction programs; to qualify for federal funds, they were also required to pass enabling legislation.(18)

Implementing the 1972 law also meant setting up multiinstitutional decision making and negotiating systems at the federal, state, and area levels. Both the federal law and the <u>Land</u> laws stipulated who was to participate in planning processes and what level of the planning process was to be involved in planning hospital resources and services.

The decision making and negotiating system for hospital planning is multilateral. Depending on the planning document that is to be produced, a different mix of governmental and nongovernmental actors interacts at the state, the regional, and the local levels. Consequently, there are elements of centralization as well as of decentralization. The complexity of the networks of governmental and nongovernmental actors defies any simple schematization. What seems clear, however, is that the actors who control planning processes retain control in spite of the participation of the central governmental hospital planners from the ministries of labor and social affairs. Also, the distribution of authority among the hospital planners and all the remaining governmental and nongovernmental actors remains the same regardless of who is participating. The hospital planners have had final decision-making authority, whereas the others have played largely consultative and advisory roles. Consequently, the participation of the hospital planners is decisive and significant in the entire process, whereas the participation of the nongovernmental actors is merely a token. The participation of the latter also seems to serve the function of reducing conflict because the participation of a large group lends support to any planning decision. To obtain support for undesirable proposals is crucial. But this system also has the effect of ensuring that those who are involved cannot complain about governmental decisions. In summary, the <u>Lander</u> are defending their powerful positions in the hospital sector not only with respect to the federal government but also with respect to other hospital-related interests.

THE AGENDA FOR FEDERAL REFORMS

In 1978 and 1979 the federal government attempted to pass legislation enbodying three goals: the improvement of the

planning and steering instruments in the hospital sector at
large; the development and application of cost-containment
measures and the introduction of economic management in
hospitals; and the strengthening of the role of insurance funds
and hospitals in the planning processes.(19) The Lander were
asked to revise existing plans of hospital needs in close
cooperation with associations of hospital and public insurance
funds in each Land. Local governments and private health
insurance interests were also to participate in this process of
revision. To serve as a criticism of ongoing hospital planning
practices, information about goals and planning criteria was to
be made available prior to final planning sessions. Drafts of
plans of hospital needs and alternative plans were to be
developed and discussed openly. Finally, governmental
hospital planners in the Land ministries were required to justify final hospital objectives, particularly in cases involving
disagreements between hospital and political interests. Except
for differences among the Lander about how to finance daily
service charges and how to interpret what final hospital goals
are to be, a considerable degree of unanimity among the
Lander has been observed in the various stages of the
legislative process from 1977 through 1979.

In late 1978, the Lander rejected the federal proposals.
They voted for the maintenance of existing practices and
mechanisms in hospital planning, for full coverage of operating
costs through hospital charges, and for pluralism in hospital
ownership. They insisted that the authority for
decision making and planning stay centralized at the state
level, rather than at the federal level and that negotiations
involving rate setting remain entirely decentralized at the local
level, that is, at the level of individual sickness funds and
hospitals. The Lander argued that local and regional
variations in the need for hospital services precluded the
application of uniform national criteria. Instead, they argued,
selective measures are required both for hospital planning and
hospital rate setting, and final authority should rest with the
Land ministries.

IMPLICATIONS FOR REFORMS

This examination of recent health-policy developments has
highlighted the state of flux in policies that affect the medical
and hospital care subsectors and the existence of relatively
stable and exclusive compulsory membership organizations that
are adapting to increasing financial and political pressures.
These quasipublic organizations are hierarchically structured
and preside over negotiations in medical care, hospital
planning, and the financing of hospital investment. The
corporate structures in the medical sector appear more stable

and exclusive than those in the sector of hospital care. However, when hospital-planning and investment-financing activities are evaluated in terms of results, the structures in the hospital sector and the dominant actors who control them seem stable and exclusive as well.

Other findings reveal the relatively high degree of sharing of legislative and regulatory authority that has been observed between the federal government and the Lander and between the bureaucracies of insurance funds and physicians' associations. Two dominant modes for financing medical and hospital care and health facilities prevail: public and private insurance and grants-in-aid programs. Sector-by-sector decision making and also intrasectoral fragmentation of responsibility provide the basic context for any reforms that are made in the health field.

Designs for the formulation and the administration of decisions about the two medical care subsectors reveal a built-in bias in favor of corporate structures, compulsory-membership organizations, and individual organizations (hospitals and local insurance funds). Individual citizen/consumers are at a distinct disadvantage. As a result of historical institutional, political, and administrative traditions, these corporate participants have favored positions.

The research makes it clear that the management of information and data systems by corporate and governmental structures at all organizational levels raises new and important issues concerning changing power relationships rather than health issues as such. These issues focus on information and data systems as tools for keeping and extending power or for making decisions. There is considerable evidence that national and subnational organizational elites use data systems as power instruments. Hence power relationships among the membership organizations of either the medical or the fund corporate structures are shifting. Relationships among levels of governmental bureaucracies also seem to be shifting. There is considerably less evidence that data and information systems are used for decision making at different organizational levels. The use of these information and data systems seem to change as one moves from the lower to the higher levels of the corporate and governmental structures. At the lower levels, they are aids used in decision making. At the upper level, they are instruments of power.

Cross-national experiences, particularly those associated with the 1974 reorganization of Britain's National Health Services and with organizational reforms effected in Sweden since 1965, teach some lessons that are worthwhile because of the potential they provide for cost-containment and for increasing citizens' influence over providers.

If the Swedish and British models for decentralizing health responsibilities, resources, and management capabilities are compared to decentralization in the Federal Republic of Germany, it is clear that Germany has no macroinstitutional infrastructures and mechanisms for accountability that match those of Sweden and Britain. In these countries, areawide and local governments are subject to some degree of accountability through elections and the delineation of administrative responsibilities. The German case differs considerably because of the mix of governmental and quasipublic institutions and of accountability structures that operate at different levels of the public policy-making system. Before any model of decentralization can work, the Federal Republic of Germany must obtain a better coordination of governmental and quasigovernmental structures and of political and administrative provisions for accountability.

Major tasks for research remain. Information is needed not only about the multilayered, subnational implementation structures, but also about the flow of finances under social insurance programs. The cumulative impact of the coexistence of governmental and insurance structures whose lines of authority and mechanisms of accountability are not the same must also be explored. The experiences of other continental European countries with similar insurance schemes may be more relevant than those of Sweden and Britain. Normative decentralization schemes that ignore financial and administrative interdependencies seem to be doomed to failure.

NOTES

1.   Theoretical and empirical literature cannot be discussed in this paper, and statistical materials and developmental data are not included. The findings reported are based on documentary analyses, on primary and secondary sources, and on numerous intensive interviews with key actors, conducted during the months of September through December of 1978 in selected subnational research sites. A mix of closed- and open-ended interview questionnaire methods was used. Subnational research sites were selected on the basis of their representativeness of similar and dissimilar circumstances of governance and of problem areas in health. They were selected on the basis of population profiles, location, resources distribution, and similar factors pertinent to generalizations about implementation of health programs in the Federal Republic of Germany.

2.   Wissentschaftliches Institut der Ortskrankenkassen, eds., Personalentwicklung im Gesundheitwesen in Vergangenheit und Zukunft (Bonn-Bad Godesberg: Wido-Materialien Band 2, 1979), pp. 32-54. The tremendous difficulties in using German health data are discussed

extensively by the authors as well as data reliability as a result of constantly changing formats, concepts, and focal interests in health statistics. Furthermore, this publication provides a balanced interpretation of data on the health-services sector and on boundary problems of the health with other services sectors.

3.   Der Bundesminister fur Jegend, Familie und Gesundheit, Daten des Gesundheitswesense-Ausgabe 1977 (Bonn-Bad Godesberg: Palatio-Druck Heitzer gmbH, 1977), pp. 239-263.   Rather than quoting numerous other sources for aggregate national data on health expenditures and cost developments, some comments should be made that have immediate and practical relevance. It is a fairly widespread practice, at least, outside the inner circle of governmental and nongovernmental specialists to discuss cost developments in the health field as an aggregate phenomenon. Therefore global decision instruments are requested to address these cost developments. Often, the interdependence of costs in one area with costs in another tends to be minimized. The interdependent impact of separate decisions on hospital investments and hospital charges - two areas of interest to this study - is much stronger than available statistics and the existence of separate decision structures in the two areas suggest. The dynamics of distinct cost developments often tend to be obscured. There is an additional problem which, unless it is accounted for, can lead to quite different interpretations. For example, if one were to analyze the annual growth rate of hospital expenditures in 1974 which was as high as 30 percent, one would insist on stringent policy instruments to prevent or reduce this growth rate to 10 percent, for example. In reality, a change in law required different accounting procedures and included different expenditure items than had been included under the previous prevailing practice. The changes in the law were reflected in available statistics in 1974 for the first time.

4.   For a good discussion of some of these problems, see Amitai Etzioni, "Societal Overload: Sources, Components, and Corrections," Political Science Quarterly, vol. 92, number 4, Winter 1977-78, pp. 607-632; and Richard Rose and Guy Peters, Can Government Go Bankrupt? (New York: Basic Books, 1978).

5.   See reference 2, p. 18.

6.   As the research focus shifts from formal to informal elements and from a national to a subnational perspective, a more fragmented system of health responsibilities appears than was suggested in the author's earlier study Health Policy Making and Administration in West Germany and the United States (Beverly Hills: Sage Publications,

1974). Detailed references to publications and studies in the Federal Republic of Germany that serve as background for this study are contained in the author's case studies on Health Planning Methods for Ambulatory Care: The Case of the Federal Republic of Germany, in Discussion Paper Series, dp./77-79 International Institute of Management, Wissenschaftszentrum-Berlin; and Hospital Planning in North Rhine Westphalia: Its Actors, Structures and Processes, in: Discussion Paper Series, dp/78-19, International Institute of Management, Wissenschaftszentrum Berlin, February 1978; see also the author's, Organizations for Managing National Hospital Planning Programs in France and the Federal Republic of Germany, [US/HEW, National Institute of Health, Bethesda, Maryland, 1979, DHEW Publication No. (NIH) 79-1494].

7.   This discovery is no surprise. Even in what seems to be a political system which is more ideologically oriented and consequently centralized, legislative goals seldom pursue one objective only. Goal ambivalence is a basic characteristic of public policy making. Even though Hugh Heclo and others are considered theoretical agnostics, their insights and explanations of policy developments over time portray a sense of historical realism and of the nature of policy making over time, missing elsewhere. For the discussion on theoretical agnosticism, see Fritz W. Scharpf, European Journal of Political Research 6 (1978): 117-125; see Hugh Heclo, Modern Social Politics in Britain and Sweden (New Haven: Yale University Press, 1974); Arnold J. Heidenheimer, Hugh Heclo, Carolyn Adams, Comparative Public Policy, The Position of Social Choice in Europe and America (New York: St. Martin's Press, 1975).

8.   For a good discussion that Selbstverwaltung may have been a fiction rather than reality historically, see Christian von Ferber, "Sociale Selbstverwaltung," vol. 1, Bonn-Duisdorf, Verlag der Ortskrankenkassen, pp. 99-199. Also, the three German national parties seem to share equally in centralization and bureaucratization processes.

9.   On the significance of symbolic actions in politics and administration, see Murray Edelman, The Symbolic Use of Politics, (Urbana: University of Illinois Press, 1964).

10.   See the analysis of the performance of two national health programs over a forty-year period by Christa Altenstetter and James W. Bjorkman, Federal-State Health Policies and Impacts: The Politics of Implementation (Washington, D.C.: University Press of America, 1978). For a comprehensive discussion of interorganizational aspects of national program implementation from a cross-national perspective, see Kenneth Hanf and Fritz W.

Scharpf, eds., Interorganizational Policy Making (London: Sage Publications, 1978), see in particular the chapter by Hanf, Hjern, and Porter.

11. Christa Altenstetter, "The Impact of Organizational Arrangements on Policy Performance," chapter 2 in Christa Altenstetter, ed., National-Subnational Relations in Health: Opportunities and Constraints [Bethesda, Maryland: National Institute of Health, 1978, DHEW Publication No. (NIH) 78-182], pp. 15-35.

12. See reference 2.

13. For a comprehensive legal discussion, see Harald Bogs, "Strukturprobleme der Selbstverwaltung einer modernen Sozialversicherung" in Harald Bogs and Christian von Ferber, Soziale Selbstverwaltung, vol. 1, Bonn-Duisdorf, Verlag der Ortskrankenkasse, pp. 13-96.

14. For a discussion of dimensions, types and theories of accountability, see James W. Bjorkman and Christa Altenstetter, "Accountability in Health Care: An Essay on Mechanisms, Muddles, and Mires," in Journal of Health Politics, Policy and Law, forthcoming in 1979.

15. Christa Altenstetter, "The Role of the Lander in Hospital Planning: The Case of the Federal Republic of Germany," chapter 11 in Altenstetter, ed., op. cit., pp. 330-356.

16. Excluded from financial support were medical schools (supported by a separate federal-state appropriation program), private, for profit hospitals, nursing homes, specialized TB-hospitals, hospitals operated by insurance funds that do not serve the population at large, rehabilitation facilities (Kur) and, finally, hospitals under 100 beds. The financing of training facilities and of accommodations for nursing and other health personnel was also excluded.

17. Deborah A. Stone, "Professionalism and Accountability: Controlling Health Services in the United States and West Germany," Journal of Health Politics, Policy and Law, vol. 2, 1977, pp. 32-47.

18. See reference 7, Hospital Planning.

19. This summary is based on the latest version of reform proposals available in early 1979. Several different versions had circulated in 1978 which ranged from "working papers" to first position papers, and finally, after numerous changes were made as a result of lobbying efforts, to the first federal bill.

15 Health Care Policy Strategies and Political Coalitions in the United States*

Lawrence D. Brown

To many observers, federal health-care policy in the United States amounts to little more than a collection of fragmented and unsystematic interventions into equally fragmented and unsystematic methods of financing health-care delivery that is loosely called "the American health-care system." This view of policy may reflect reality or it may reflect a failure to discern the method behind the apparent madness.

Federal health-care policy is less imperfectly developed than is usually assumed. The federal government has intervened in the health-care system by means of four strategies, each of which has emerged as a response to the perceived weaknesses of the previous one and each of which is based upon a distinct rationale. Moreover, each of these strategies is employed in a distinct political "arena," and each embraces distinct political coalitions. Analyzing these strategy arenas is essential to understanding the behavior of the federal government in the health-care field and to explaining, evaluating, and predicting policy outcomes.

*This is a revised version of a paper prepared for a Conference on Participation and Policy Making, Adademie fur Politische Bildung, Tutzing, Federal Republic of Germany, June 5-9, 1978. Views expressed here should not be attributed to the Brookings Institution, to its trustees, officers, or other staff members.

FOUR STRATEGIES OF INTERVENTION

Federal government pursues four major types of activities in the health-care field:

1. Government may <u>subsidize</u> the health-care system. Government may also offer grants-in-aid to health-care providers and institutions to do more of what they are presently doing or more of what they would like to be doing. The major examples are federal support for National Institutes of Health (NIH) biomedical research; Hill-Burton program for the planning, construction, renovation, and expansion of medical facilities; and federal aid for the training of physicians and other medical personnel.

2. Government may intervene in the <u>financing</u> of health-care, usually by authorizing funds that entitle individuals to care at least partly at public expense. Obvious examples are Medicare and Medicaid.

3. Government may <u>reorganize</u> the delivery system. As a rule, reorganization involves an effort to add new organizational forms to existing ones. Cases in point are neighborhood or community health centers; health-maintenance organizations (HMOs) and National Health Service Corps (NHSC).

4. Government may impose planning, coordination, and/or <u>regulation</u> on the delivery system. It may do this in connection with financing programs or independently of them. Examples are comprehensive health-planning (CHP) agencies, which were transformed into health-systems agencies (HSAs) under the Health Resources Planning and Development Act of 1974; professional standards review organizations (PSROs); and certificate-of-need programs, initiated by the states, but now required of all states by the federal government.

STRATEGIES AS POLICY RESPONSES

As the federal role in American health care has grown, the four strategies of intervention have come to prominence roughly in sequence, each taking precedence as the others showed themselves to be limited or to have failed.

As the nation emerged from World War II, many observers believed that American health care suffered above all from a shortage of resources - a shortage of doctors, of hospitals, and of biomedical knowledge. The federal subsidy programs that emerged - NIH project grants, Hill-Burton formula grants, and grants of various types for medical schools - were intended to remedy this shortage.

By the mid-1960s, the "more-is-better" approach was increasingly challenged. Just as general economic growth could not guarantee cures for unemployment and poverty, it became clear that continuous additions to the number of "inputs" in the existing system could not by themselves guarantee access to adequate medical care for the elderly and the poor. A federal role in financing medical care seemed to be the answer, and the government assumed that role in Medicare and Medicaid.

By 1970, the infusion of large new federal funds into the delivery system had produced both severe inflation and growing doubts about the appropriateness of the care being purchased. In 1973, after three years of debate, the federal government decided to initiate a reshaping of the system itself. Health Maintenance Organizations (HMOs), launched and supported with federal grants and loans, were to cut costs, shake up the traditional fee-for-service sector by means of market competition, and make new care available to the underserved.

It very soon became clear, however, that for many reasons HMOs would prove to be a solution that was too little and too late. Regulation, long a watchword of health planners and critics, became a reality as federal law supported professional standards review-organizations, health-systems agencies, certificate-of-need measures, and state rate-setting experiments.

Thus, the federal presence in the health-care system has grown. In each phase of the growth of intervention there was a dominant strategic approach. In each case, time, experience, and reflection produced challenges to the dominant strategy. In each case, the federal government responded by adopting new strategies designed to address new priorities and by reordering priorities.

ARENAS AND COALITIONS

It may be argued that the four health-care strategies summarized above correspond to four political arenas in which political processes take place. The term arena is meant to denote a policy subsystem in which the participants play roles that are relatively stable over time and significantly different from roles they (and other participants) play in other subsystems.

For present purposes, a coalition is two or more political actors who together work for a policy proposal. Actors are found within institutions, of which five are of central importance to this analysis of federal health policy: the Executive branch, Congress, the federal bureaucracy, interest groups, and state and local governments.(1) These institutions are obviously not internally homogeneous: Each contains many actors. Some form coalitions with others and some never coalesce with others on a policy position. Coalition-building takes place both within and between institutions. If sufficient agreement cannot be reached within one or more institutions, coalition building may be blocked. If sufficient agreement cannot be reached among most of these institutions, coalition building is very likely to fail. (Only the president and Congress hold veto power; all five of these institutions wield influence, however.)

The rationale behind the subsidy strategy was conservative. What the system needed, the subsidy advocates maintained, was additions to the supply of medical resources and services. The system was basically sound; what was needed was more of it. Additions to the stock of biomedical knowledge, hospitals, and manpower would trickle down to the poor and out of the hinterlands. The strategy was based on comfortable assumptions and for about twenty years generated little controversy or resistance. The American Medical Association (AMA) supported hospital construction and did not oppose NIH research. The subsidy programs imposed no costs on organized groups and offered a range of benefits, both specific and general. Specifically, the research community, hospital administrators and trustees, medical students, and others gained tangibly from these programs. More generally, those longing for a cure to cancer, heart disease, and other diseases - that is, the whole population - identified with and endorsed these programs, too. These programs met in very high degree the conditions of a sucessful coalition: they diffused costs broadly; they offered specific benefits to a sizable number of watchful and activated groups; and they promised broad social benefits with which most of the population could identify.

The impetus for the subsidy programs did not come from the executive. President Harry S. Truman had identified himself closely with the abortive fight for national health insurance (NHI) in the late forties, and the subsidy programs were not high on his list of priorities. Some congressmen, however, perceived that a subsidy approach was far less controversial than NHI and that it was likely to be highly popular. For this reason most congressmen remained supportive but detached, happy to defer to the leadership of the chairman of the Labor-HEW subcommittees of the appropriate committees.

These patterns define the politics of the subsidy arena: limited interest-group opposition; strong interest-group support; diffused costs combined with many specific and general benefits; a nonideological, nonpartisan and un-controversial character; relatively weak executive interest;

and widespread but detached congressional support. For twenty years, the subsidy strategy was the health-care policy of the federal government.

By the middle 1960s, the subsidy arena's privileged "triple alliance" politics came increasingly under assault.(2) NIH was exposed to growing skepticism as the legislative committees, following the general trend toward short-term authorizations, cast a closer look on its activities; as investigative committees cast aspersions on the Institutes' management; as critics - including President Richard M. Nixon - wondered aloud whether NIH was up to waging a "war on cancer";(3) as a natural question - where, after the great promise and twenty years of generous funding, are the "cures" for cancer, heart disease, and the rest? - was asked more insistently; as disputes about the relative merits of basic versus applied research grew more acerbic; and as the notion that personal prevention, not a sudden biomedical cure, was perhaps the best means of avoiding cancer took hold in the popular mind. The cumulative result was a growing willingness of Congress, the Executive branch, and the public to challenge NIH's priorities, activities, and management.

At about the same time that criticism of NIH was growing, Hill-Burton became the focus of a debate between rural spokesmen and rural congressmen, whose districts had been the main beneficiaries of the program for twenty years, and urban spokesmen and congressmen, who argued that the cities' need to build new outpatient facilities and to modernize obsolete hospitals far outweighed the rural areas' need to build new hospitals. As evidence accumulated that many parts of the nation had an overabundance of beds and that this excess of beds fueled the inflation of medical cost, the urban interests succeeded in transforming the program to benefit them more.(4)

The medical manpower-training programs, enacted later, also were challenged. By the early 1970s, policy analysts and many congressmen were convinced that the nation's medical manpower problem was not an overall doctor shortage, but rather a shortage of certain types of doctors in certain areas. Abandoning the view that more is better, Congress began attaching strings to manpower-training awards to encourage the growth of a larger supply of family practitioners and to favor underserved areas.(5) By 1978, Joseph Califano, Secretary of HEW in the Carter administration, was arguing publicly that the nation suffered from a surplus of physicians which drove costs up severely.(6)

Congress is not likely to end these subsidy programs soon.(7) However, the strains that have beset the once tranquil subsidy coalitions have robbed them of their earlier sacrosanct status and have subjected them, along with more run-of-the-mill programs, to public controversy and debate. The strains have also slowed the growth of their budgets.(8)

Momentum toward some form of national health insurance has ebbed and flowed in the United States since the New Deal.(9) Unlike the subsidy strategy, however, financing proposals have evoked intense interest-group conflict. The AFL-CIO has led the support, which has been countered by strong, indeed vehement, opposition by the AMA. Unlike the nonpartisan subsidy programs, moreover, financing has been highly partisan: In the postwar period, Democratic presidents (Truman, Kennedy, Johnson, and Carter) have all made public commitments to NHI; the Republican presidents (Eisenhower, Nixon, and Ford) have made no sustained initiatives toward it. The program's dollar costs would be diffused, but proposals threatened specific groups - doctors, hospitals, and insurance firms - with possibly radical changes in their modes of business. Benefits would accrue more narrowly than those of the subsidy programs; they would go to the elderly and the poor, for instance. Controversial, ideological, and partisan, NHI proposals split Congress into several blocs.

By the early 1960s, some form of NHI appeared imminent. It was widely conceded that problems in the health-care system would not automatically fade as the supply of resources and services increased. Older and poorer citizens, in particular, faced serious financial obstacles to obtaining health care, and there was a resultant demand for direct government intervention. The problem, however, was to find a legislative solution on which contending ideological and partisan blocs could agree.

Whereas the characteristics of the subsidy arena were ideally suited to congressional leadership, the divisiveness of financing issues precluded it. Financing politics begin in earnest when the executive sets them in motion. Thus, the first step in coalition building for medicare involved developing a plausible executive initiative. The task fell to HEW.(10) By the early 1960s, NHI proponents were convinced that the wisest course was to propose federal support by means of the social security system (which conferred the legitimacy of contributions, contracts, and rights on what might otherwise appear to be a "handout" program) to cover hospital bills (which were the most expensive and least inclined to upset physicians over federal intrusion into their private practices) of the elderly (a group which evoked considerable sympathy and whose bills fell on a large share of the population - that is, on their children).

The second step called for congressional participation. In the medicare struggle, the main scene of action was the House Ways and Means Committee, headed by Wilbur Mills (D-Ark.), a legislator highly respected for substantive expertise and political sagacity. Used to dealing with highly partisan legislation, Ways and Means had developed methods for

reconciling that gave major committee and interest-group
factions a share of the outcome for which they might claim
credit and that took careful account of the mood of the House
as a whole.(11)   Seeking to build a supportive coalition and to
anticipate problems at the roll-call stage on the floor, Mills
altered the Johnson administration's proposal significantly by
adding Medicare Part B (a voluntary program financed by
subscriber premiums and general revenues to cover physicians'
services for the elderly) and a Medicaid program (which gave
federal matching funds to the states to support medical
payments for public-assistance recipients).(12)

The third stage required marshalling a majority of votes
in both House and Senate to pass the revised measure.   A
proposal was ready, congressional leadership was newly willing
to "perfect" the bill as a result of the new composition of the
Congress, and the votes were at hand.   The long struggle for
NHI culminated in an explosion of support for Medicare and
Medicaid in 1965.

With the advent of these new programs, the federal
government simultaneously funded increases in both the supply
of medical resources and services and in the demand for them,
and it did so in a medical marketplace subject to peculiar and
highly inflationary tendencies.   Moreover, it pursued this
course without significant controls or costs.   Medicare and
Medicaid legislation gave recipients an entitlement to care,
thereby committing the government to pay without budgetary
limit the bills recipients incurred.   Nor were meaningful controls placed on the behavior of the provider: In the debate
over the programs, fee schedules had been mentioned in
passing; but no one wanted to antagonize organized medicine
even further and open up new confounding questions that
might have jeopardized passage of the bill.(13)   Since controls
on either providers or consumers were lacking, Medicare and
Medicaid costs quickly soared.   The federal government had
become a major purchaser of care and was purchasing from a
highly disadvantageous position.   A major watershed had been
reached, one that altered the stakes of coalition building
decisively.

The third kind of strategy, reorganization, involves a
federal effort to change the cast of characters in the
health-care system.   In the United States any proposal that
dramatically upsets or displaces established organizations faces
severe political handicaps.   For this reason, health-policy
reorganization efforts almost always involve a public effort to
launch new organizations and add them, preferably incon-
spicuously, to the existing system.

Because the political costs usually equal or outweigh the
benefits, reorganization efforts tend to be encapsulated in
small project grant efforts at the periphery of federal
health-care programs.   In one important case, however - the

health-maintenance organization - a reorganization program came to center stage. The origins and progress of this program demonstrate the basic character of the reorganization arena.(14)

In 1970, top HEW officials in the Nixon administration were anxiously casting about for a new approach that would brake rising Medicare and Medicaid costs to the government and deflect attention from the movement, led by congressional Democrats, for NHI. The HEW generalists were delighted when Dr. Paul Ellwood explained and extolled the virtues of a federal effort to create prepaid group-practice plans, which he called "health maintenance organizations."(15) HMOs, obliged to operate within a fixed budget, able to exceed that budget only at the risk of imposing a premium increase on subscribers the next year, constrained by the need to compete with established insurance plans, and (as a result of all this) required to absorb the increases in their costs instead of passing them along to third parties, reversed the illogical incentives for fee-for-service practice. Moreover - a very important point to the worried generalists - if HMOs became sufficiently popular and widespread, the federal government would be able to purchase care for Medicare and Medicaid beneficiaries for fixed fees known in advance, thereby introducing a measure of control into uncontrollable federal spending. In 1971, the HMO approach won enthusiastic, explicit presidential endorsement when Nixon called for a program of grants and loans to launch prepaid practice plans around the nation, especially in underserved areas.(16)

The coalition-building process that led to enactment of HMO legislation in 1973 displayed the distinctive features of post-Medicare politics. As coalitions formed around the proposal it became clear that a federal HMO policy agreeable to all major interests would be difficult, perhaps impossible, to create. The Nixon initiative was extraordinary in itself: A conservative Republican president offered legislation that would save public money by challenging the Republican party's staunchest and wealthiest supporters, organized doctors. The proposal, which defined HMOs in very broad and inclusive terms, also offended purists in the prepaid group-practice movement.(17) The proposal also offended congressional Democrats, who saw that the vagueness of the Nixon bill would allow HEW, and therefore the administration itself, to define and shape HMOs virtually as they chose. Both groups agreed that the bill should be redrawn in Congress to include many specifics and safeguards.

This alliance soon broke down, however, over precisely what the specifics and safeguards should be. Some conservative and moderate legislators, heavily represented on the health subcommittee of the House Interstate and Foreign Commerce Committee, viewed HMOs mainly as an interesting but

limited   experiment   in   market-oriented,   incentive-based
techniques of cost-containment. Some liberals, notably Senator
Edward M. Kennedy (D-Mass.), chairman of the health
subcommittee of the Labor and Public Welfare Committee (now
called "Human Resources") thought that federal support for
HMOs could be justified only if the new plans corrected many
of the inadequacies and inequities of fee-for-service medicine
and conventional insurance. To win liberal support, HMOs had
to do more and do it better. Thus, Kennedy wanted HMOs to
provide a wide, indeed comprehensive, range of health-care
benefits.
     The agreement finally reached with the enactment of the
Health Maintenance Organization Act in December 1972 pleased
none of the major participants. It required HMOs to practice
community rating and to hold an open enrollment period; in
both cases, subsidy provisions were replaced by grants of
administrative discretion so that HEW could help plans which
the requirements might damage. The HMO community damned
the law as unworkable.
     HEW made repeated efforts to write regulations that were
at once responsible to the language and intent of the law and
responsive   to   the   preferences   of   the   HMOs,   but   none
succeeded. Under pressure from HMO spokesmen, Congress
amended the law in 1976 and 1978, but by early 1979, more than
five years after enactment of the law and after almost a decade
of federal HMO promotion, the results were hardly impressive.
Only about 80 HMOs had "qualified" under the law as amended,
less than 4 percent of the population belonged to one, and
almost half of this 4 percent lived in California.(18)   Part -
probably most - of the problem has little to do with the federal
government.   HMOs   are   extremely   complex   organizations,
difficult to build and sustain in the best of circumstances, that
run against deeply rooted patterns in the American health-care
system. That the federal government has proved unable to
reduce the obstacles is, in turn, largely explained by the fact
that   political   coalition-building   in   the   HMO   program   never
stabilized. The major participants have never been able to
agree on what the elusive legislative hybrid, the "federally
qualified HMO," ought to be.
     The fourth strategy of intervention is regulation, a direct
declaration by public authorities about what providers (and/or
consumers) may or may not do. The existence of political
efforts to regulate health care is problematic, for regulation
requires that direct, tangible, salient costs be imposed on
organized and self-conscious groups and institutions in order
to confer indirect, untraceable, and marginal benefits on an
unorganized   and   inattentive   general   public.   Unlike   the
subsidy, regulation does not contribute to the search for the
cure of disease; indeed it may curb technological innovation
and diffusion. It builds no beds and trains no doctors.

Regulation does not, like the financing programs, expand purchasing power and economic access to care for large numbers of voters. It does not even promise creative, progressive experiments in health-care delivery, as do reorganization efforts. For the most part, regulation involves constraining.

True, everyone benefits from lower health-related taxes, insurance premiums, and out-of-pocket costs. However, cost-containment is more likely to produce a deceleration of cost increases than an absolute decrease and saving. Nor is this deceleration - assuming that it is perceived and considered significant by large numbers of the public - likely to be clearly traceable to regulatory programs. When the political credit claimed for saving money is counterbalanced by the arguments of providers that the government has regulated them into offering inferior quality and limited access, the perceived public - and political - benefits of the regulatory arena seem dim indeed. For these and other reasons, many informed political scientists could have explained in 1970 why the federal government was quite unlikely to attempt to regulate health care in the near future. Yet in 1972, the government authorized Professional Standard Review Organizations (PSROs) to review the need for and appropriateness of hospital admissions and lengths-of-stay in certain federal programs. In 1974, it set up Health Systems Agencies (HSAs) to draw up short-term and long-term plans for allocation of resources within defined geographic areas. At the same time, it required that those states without certificate-of-need laws adopt them. The government has also supported endeavors by states to set rates.

Coalitions in support of health-care regulation depend upon three rationales; (19) each may be entertained by individuals who have little faith in the others. The first rationale is that the federal government's post-Medicare position as a major purchaser of health care confers on it responsibilities more demanding than those it should fulfill in other areas of social policy whose commodities it purchases less extensively. Since the enactment of Medicare and Medicaid, the federal budget has become a major source of health-care dollars. This situation has made budget makers of the Executive and in Congress nervous, and is also generally recognized as a major cause of increased taxes, insurance premiums, and out-of-pocket health-care costs. The federal government's new role and responsibilities in health-care financing have led some fiscal conservatives to reconsider their normal aversion to federal regulation. (20)

A second rationale for regulation centers on the peculiar nature of the health-care market. Although the precise extent and nature of market imperfections in health care are endlessly debatable, policy makers tend to perceive and deplore one

imperfection above others: the perverse tendency for health
costs to rise as a result not of <u>under</u>supply of resources and
services but rather as a result of <u>over</u>supply.   By the early
1970s, the arguments of health planners that an overabundance
of hospital beds, procedures, technology, and certain kinds of
specialists - notably surgeons - was contributing steadily to
cost escalation had taken hold.   The federal government was
not only underwriting large new increases in demand but also
was simultaneously subsidizing expansion of unneeded, expensive, and cost-generating resources.   Recognition of this
seemingly egregious waste prodded sizable numbers of liberals
and conservatives toward providing means of controlling the
supply.

Third,   regulation   appealed   to   critics   of   prevailing
practices who wanted to introduce planning, coordination, and
regulation into the system to rationalize it, and to reduce the
dominance   of   individual   and   organized   providers   over
resources.   The liberals' desire was not new, but when it
combined with regulatory rationales appealing to conservatives
and moderates in new and special post-Medicare conditions, the
core of a coalition was formed.

In   short,   the   basis   for   a   potent   potential   regulatory
coalition   did   exist   beneath   the   superficially   unreceptive
political surface.   Realizing the potential of this coalition,
however,   depends   upon   reaching   practical   and   detailed
agreement   among   very   diverse   viewpoints   on   acceptable
<u>mechanisms</u> of regulation.   A look at the lawmakers' options
shows   why   decentralized   regulation   has   emerged   as   the
preferred mode.

Basically,   three   approaches   were   open   to   the   policy
makers.   First, they could attempt to write carefully worded
regulatory <u>laws</u>.   This approach was unattractive for several
reasons.   First, members of the regulatory coalition were not
sure what their operational goals were, and they knew that
they   would   start   to   quarrel   as   soon   as   they   got   down   to
detail.   Moreover, the political stakes were too low to justify a
great investment of time, effort, mental exercise, and staff
energies.   It was also clear that the things to be regulated -
"quality" of care, "need" for expanded hospital facilities,
"necessity" for admission to hospitals, and so forth - are
extremely difficult to define, must be explained differently in
different circumstances, and cannot be defined in intelligent
detail in a statute written in Washington.   These obstacles
persuaded   the   executive   and   Congress   alike   that   detailed
regulatory legislation was not a workable approach.

Second, a different approach to central regulation could
have been taken.   Strong regulatory powers could have been
conferred on the federal bureaucracy.   This approach, too,
was unappealing.   Congressional conservatives and top officials
in the Nixon and Ford administrations, wedded to the concept

of "new federalism," did not want to increase the powers of social planner bureaucrats or to encourage highhanded federal bureaucratic dictation. By the same token, liberal Democrats in Congress did not wish to invest secretaries of HEW in conservative Republican administrations with strong regulatory powers. Moreover, liberals and conservatives in Congress and the Executive alike could see that the health units of HEW were too disorganized, chaotic, and fragmented to be suitable for a wide-ranging regulatory role. Finally, the disadvantages of preempting, in Washington, local decisions made under extremely variable conditions militated against this approach, just as they did against regulatory statutes. The barriers to legislative and administrative regulation apparently exhausted the interest of the Nixon and Ford administrations, ideologically hostile to federal regulation in any case, in taking the initiative, and they did not take it.

A third option existed, however, one likely to appeal to, and quite capable of being developed by, the legislature. This option was to set up state and local bodies, public or private, with federal sanction, aid, and guidelines, and then delegate regulatory decision making to them. This option promised the best political outcome available under the circumstances. Liberals could point to a nationwide network of organizations planning, coordinating, and challenging providers. Conservatives could rejoice in the dominant role of state and local bodies and the limited role of the federal bureaucracy. Localities could do their own planning. Interest groups would do battle at the state and local levels, not in Washington. Congressmen need not legislate in detail; they needed merely to sketch out the rudiments of a network of local organizations, leaving the details to be worked out at the local level with general guidance from HEW. Antagonism over the inevitable frictions of regulation would fall upon state and local participants, not on federal policy makers. For these reasons, decentralization and delegation became the major federal watch-words in the developing regulatory arena.

The explanation of the appeal of decentralized regulation lies in the nature of the coalition-building task. A coalition that would pull apart over the substance of regulation could maintain agreement over regulatory procedures and structures. Delegation of regulatory authority dealt with widely perceived problems, but absolved the federal government of responsibility. Sketching out a general approach while leaving detailed, operational decisions to state and local regulators permitted a small number of congressmen - those unconcerned about cost-containment and waste and those not eager to introduce planning and rationality into the system - to come together, win the acquiescence of a sizable number of less committed legislators, claim credit for federal initiatives emphasizing economizing or planning, and leave the hard, unpopular decisions to state and local authorities.

Many observers doubt that a decentralized approach to health-care regulation can work. State and local regulators may be too close to, and too intimately involved in, the settled expectations of communities of consumers and providers to make and hold firm, unpopular decisions under pressure. Regulation must address itself to two types of areas in the United States: underserved ones that want more resources and services and adequately served ones that want to stay that way or get even better service. Nay-saying and limitation become extremely difficult in these circumstances, especially for area representatives or officials accountable to area representatives. Perhaps for these reasons, the Carter administration proposed a more centralized approach in 1977.(21) To date, however, Congress, the architect of the decentralized regulatory approach, has resisted the administration's appeal for a federally imposed limit on hospital revenues and expansion funds.

THE COHERENCE OF POLICY: INCONSISTENCY OF INSTITUTIONALIZED AMBIVALENCE?

Although the four strategies of Federal intervention emerged sequentially, each being in some measure an effort to supplement earlier ones, the effort at rationalization, ironically, has itself produced a steady complication and fragmentation of federal health-care programs. With two strategies the government encourages growth in the supply of and demand for resources and services. With two others, the government simultaneously tries to constrain growth in the supply of and demand for resources and services.

There is also much to fault in the individual strategies themselves. In the subsidy arena, the federal government gives generous support to providers having for more than twenty years asked few questions about the promise of biomedical breakthroughs, the costs of unconstrained diffusion of medical technology, and the need for and costs of new hospital construction and expansion. The financing programs created promised care to many consumers and then reimbursed providers their "reasonable and customary" fees without much concern for the financial consequences. Reorganization efforts have had little impact on the larger system, and regulatory efforts, although they have not had time to prove themselves, may be too decentralized and lacking in sanctions to bring costs under control.

Significant federal involvement in the health-care system, however, is little more than thirty years old. The major turning point in political attitudes and constraints - resulting in the development of Medicare and Medicaid - came only a

decade and a half ago, and the federal government began
experimenting in earnest with controls only within the last
seven years. Wavering and inelegant policy-making politics in
the United States have produced a great deal of activity in
remarkably short periods of time.

Far from being static and deadlocked, federal health-care
policy has been, since the enactment of Medicare, remarkably
innovative and responsive. Since 1970, the government has
moved rapidly into areas - reorganization and regulation - that
were an anathema to it a few years earlier. Most of the
priorities about which the system's critics contend the federal
government should be "doing something" are in fact being
addressed in some manner.

PROSPECTS AND CONCLUSIONS:
TOWARD CENTRALIZATION, AMERICAN STYLE

Today the politics of federal health-care policy are
temporarily at rest, awaiting the formation of new coalitions to
extend or amend past policies and to alter the policy mix. It
is possible that a crossroads has been reached that is
comparable in importance to the enactment of Medicare and
Medicaid, which changed the federal role substantially by
making the central government a major purchaser of care and
thereby launching the quest for controls that introduced new
reorganization and regulatory strategies. Today, as activity
proceeds in all four arenas, new questions about the federal
role are being raised, and the interplay between politics and
policy may be entering a new stage.

The most important feature of the United States political
system is its extensive structural decentralization, meaning its
heavy reliance on the private sector in collective decision
making, its broad delegations of power to state and local
governments, and its wide separation of powers among
executives, legislatures, and courts at all levels of
government. Not surprisingly, strategy has tended to follow
structure. The most prominent feature of the federal
health-care efforts reviewed here has been the repeated
resorting to decentralized strategies to achieve the central
government's ends. Federal involvement in the health-care
system has subsidized, matched, entitled, catalyzed, or
delegated responsibilities to private actors (through NIH
grants, manpower training, Medicare, HMOs, PSROs, for
example) or state and local governments (through Hill-Burton,
Medicaid, HSAs, certificate-of-need laws, and rate-setting, for
instance). This policy of decentralization honors, and flows
directly from, the structural decentralization of the United
States political system. The costs and limitations of the

approach are increasingly evident, however. The key policy questions of the coming years are likely to focus on the limitations of decentralized federal intervention, and the main political struggles of the near future will probably occur over halting and incremental efforts to widen the federal government's role in all four strategy arenas, but most especially in financing and regulation.

The federal government has four options for future policy which are illustrated by the following chart.

	Market	Regulation
Decentralized	1	2
Centralized	4	3

(1) Decentralized market solutions include efforts that work at the local level by means of money incentives and market competition to contain costs. They usually fall within the reorganization arena; the leading example is the HMO program. (2) Decentralized regulatory solutions are efforts to invest powers in public authorities at the state and local levels to allow or disallow actions of health-care providers. Examples include the four decentralized regulatory programs mentioned earlier. (3) Centralized regulation denotes federal government efforts to prescribe the behavior of health-care providers. An example is the Carter administration's proposal that Congress impose an annual 9 percent ceiling on the hospitals' capital expansion. (4) Centralized market approaches embrace federal law or regulations that attempt to influence provision or consumption of care indirectly by manipulating money and market incentives. Examples would include changes in tax laws governing deductions for medical spending, or changes in the deductibles, copayments, or premiums in the Medicare program. Centralized market approaches generally fall within the financing arena.

Some health-care economists, having persuaded themselves that all public regulation, whatever its origin, time, place or circumstance, obeys "general laws" which can be extracted from the literature on the independent regulatory commissions in Washington, argue passionately for market solutions of a financing and reorganizing nature as "alternatives" to regulation. These arguments are unlikely to prevail, however. The major forces in the health-care system -- consumer expectations, technology, physicians, hospitals, and third-party payers -- behave and interact in complex, interdependent patterns that combine market and nonmarket considerations in little-understood ways. The problem is probably not that markets are "underused" in the health-care system but instead that, given the heterogeneity of actors, forces, and motives and the interdependence among them, health-care markets operate and can only operate partially and poorly. For these reasons, few policy makers find it creditable that more extensive resort to market mechanisms will achieve the optimal and efficient ends claimed theoretically on their behalf. And even if these "alternatives" were more persuasive on the merits, there is little chance that they would emerge intact and as intended from the tortuous politics of the financing and reorganization arenas.

The economists' ardor has convinced some social scientists and journalists that today's major policy issue is the choice between markets versus regulation. This formulation is quite alien to most policy makers, however. Market forces will, for better or worse, continue to play a prominent, though partial, role in the health-care system, and the role of regulation will continue to grow. The key questions, therefore, concern the appropriate degree of centralization "versus" decentralization in both market and regulatory approaches and the proper mix between the two approaches. For reasons noted above - limited federal leverage over work-related health coverage in the private sector and federal unwillingness to make Medicare and Medicaid more "second class" than they must inevitably be - centralized market approaches are unlikely to come to center stage in the cost-containment efforts.(22) For reasons also discussed above - the difficult "technology" of organization-building efforts and lack of agreement on what organizations such as HMOs should be and do - decentralized market efforts are likely to remain peripheral too. Thus, the main center of activity is likely to be the regulatory arena, and the main practical policy choice, between decentralized and more centralized programs.

The political logic behind the current decentralized regulatory efforts was explored above. President Carter's call in 1977 for federally-imposed revenue and capital expenditure ceilings on hospitals may be a political milestone: a major far-reaching central regulatory option was placed squarely on the federal agenda for the first time. Although the 95th Congress rejected the proposal it will be debated anew in the 96th Congress. Assuming that medical cost inflation does not abate, some variant on it may well be adopted soon.(23)

The trend, in sum, appears to favor gradual, partial, but steady increases in the role of the central government in both allocating benefits and controlling costs. This trend will probably elicit increasingly derisive commentary from the growing community of policy analysts, many of whom prefer to the present melange either an effort to unleash the vigor of market forces and/or state and local governments or the introduction of "real" centralization in the European fashion where financing responsibilities fall to the central government and where costs are controlled by means of negotiations among providers, sick funds, and government over fee schedules and other administrative matters.(24) Among journalists, "attentive elites," and - for all one knows - policy makers and the general public, these insistent critiques may substantially discredit the politics of health-care policy making as they are now practiced.

A political scientist - at any rate, this political scientist - may see another side to the story, however. The prevailing approach, which constitutes a characteristically American compromise between extremes, is closely tailored to United States political and social structures. It is - or at any rate ought to be - a truism that between a policy problem and its solution political institutions always intervene. The proposals of policy analysts must be judged against the capacity of the political system to generate and implement them in something like their recommended condition, against their ability to survive the "intervening variable" of political structure.

Viewed in this light, European analogies may be little superior to market alternatives. Political fragmentation in the United States is much greater than in most European nations. In Europe, organized and articulate social strata tend to form the core of political parties; and political parties may become governments or parts of governments. In the United States, the parties are composed of relatively unorganized and often inarticulate groups that can seldom be described as "strata." Presidential and congressional nominations and elections are separate and independent processes. The executive and legislative branches may be divided between the two major parties (as they were from 1969-1976), and the parties do not "constitute" or "run" the government anyway. These institutional separations, combined with the thoroughgoing privatism and highly-valued federalism in the United States, define a degree of political decentralization unlike anything found in Europe, and greatly limit the nation's capacity to generate and implement European arrangements. In the United States, political structure and policy formation are bridged by ad hoc coalition building. This approach both presupposes and reinforces the norm that a successful outcome offers something to everyone. No group expects to win all or even most of its preferences, but all expect a share in the outcome. Judged abstractly against the economist's criteria of efficiency and the planner's standards of rationality, this norm and its outcomes may appear deficient. Judged concretely against the tendencies and capacities of United States political structure, however, the politics of federal health-care policy making may appear less peculiar; they may seem, indeed, peculiarly correct.

NOTES

(1) Institutional generalizations which this essay supports
     but does not develop may be found in Lawrence D.
     Brown, "The Formulation of Federal Health Care Policy,"
     Bulletin of the New York Academy of Medicine, vol. 54
     (January 1978), pp. 45-48.
(2) For discussion of the specifics in this paragraph, see
     Strickland, chaps. 8-10, and Natalie Davis Spingarn,
     Heartbeat: The Politics of Health Research (Washington-
     New York: Robert B. Luce, 1976).
(3) See Richard A. Rettig, Cancer Crusade: The Story of
     the National Cancer Act of 1971 (Princeton, N.J.:
     Princeton University Press, 1977).
(4) For summaries of the legislative battles, see Congres-
     sional Quarterly Almanac (CQA), 1970, p. 221 and CQA,
     1972, pp. 528-529. For background see Judith R. Lave
     and Lester B. Lave, The Hospital Construction Act: An
     Evaluation of the Hill-Burton Program, 1948-1973 (Wash-
     ington: American Enterprises Institute for Public Policy
     Research, 1974).
(5) See John K. Iglehart, "Congress Ties Medical Education
     Aid to Mandatory Increase in Enrollment," National
     Journal, October 16, 1971, pp. 2106-2107, and "Ford
     Shuns Advice in Signing New Health Manpower Bill,"
     ibid., October 23, 1976, p. 1513.
(6) U.S. Department of Health, Education, and Welfare,
     "Remarks of Joseph A. Califano, Jr., Secretary, U.S.
     Department of Health Education, and Welfare, Before the
     Association of American Medical Colleges, New Orleans,
     Louisiana, October 24, 1978." The "first tenet" of federal
     policy in the manpower training area, Califano said, is
     that "overall, we face in the next decade an oversupply
     of doctors." (p. 5) In the Carter health-care budget
     submitted to Congress a few months later, manpower-
     training programs were, as one account put it, "the big
     losers." The proposed budget would cut federal dollars
     for medical manpower training in half, eliminating al-
     together general "capitalization" grants to medical schools,
     but increasing funds for programs that require students
     to work in medically underserved areas in return for
     federal support. Congressional Quarterly Weekly Report,
     January 27, 1979, pp. 128, 120.
(7) To date, Hill-Burton suffered only a slight close call
     when Nixon vetoed its reauthorization in 1970. Congress
     reversed the veto, however, by votes of 279-98 in the
     House and 76-19 in the Senate, the first time in ten years
     that it had overturned a presidential veto. CQA 1970,
     pp. 221-228. The Nixon and Ford administrations con-

tinued to urge that the program be ended. Congress,
having shifted the program's priorities away from new
hospital construction and toward renovation of obsolete
units and construction of outpatient facilities, kept it
alive. In 1974 the program was incorporated in the new
state-centered planning process established by the Health
Resources Planning and Development Act.

(8) Hill-Burton construction support suffered most: Its
     federal outlays in constant dollars were cut roughly in
     half between fiscal year 1969 and 1975. In the middle
     and late 1960s, the NIH budget grew slowly and at times
     declined. After enactment of the National Cancer Act of
     1971, however, growth revived, especially in the cancer
     and heart institutes, which accounted for 35 percent of
     all NIH research funds in 1969, but consumed nearly 50
     percent in 1975. Manpower training budgets grew
     steadily until fiscal year 1973 and tapered off thereafter.
     Louise B. Russell and Carol S. Burke, "The Political
     Economy of Federal Health Programs in the United States:
     An Historical Review," International Journal of Health
     Services, vol. 8 (1978), pp. 61, 63, 65. See also
     Strickland, Politics, Science, and Dread Disease, pp. 212,
     313 n.19; and note 13 above.

(9) See Daniel S. Hirshfield, The Lost Reform: The Campaign
     for Compulsory Health Insurance in the United States from
     1932 to 1943 (Cambridge, Mass.: Harvard University
     Press, 1970).

(10) See Theodore R. Marmor, The Politics of Medicare
     (Chicago: Aldine, 1973), upon which this section relies
     heavily. Also useful are: Eugene Feingold, Medicare:
     Policy and Politics (San Francisco: Chandler Publishing
     Co., 1966), especially Part III; Robert J. Myers,
     Medicare (Homewood, Illinois: 1969); Richard Harris,
     A Sacred Trust (Baltimore: Penguin Books, 1969); James
     L. Sundquist, Politics and Policy: The Eisenhower,
     Kennedy, and Johnson Years (Washington: Brookings,
     1968), pp. 287-321; and Robert Stevens and Rosemary
     Stevens, Welfare Medicine in America: A Case Study of
     Medicaid (New York: The Free Press, 1974).

(11) John F. Manley, The Politics of Finance: The House
     Committee on Ways and Means (Boston: Little, Brown,
     1970) and Fenno, Congressmen in Committees, passim.

(12) Marmor, The Politics of Medicare, pp. 60-70.

(13) Ibid., pp. 71-72.

(14) The account of HMO politics presented here draws upon
     the author's manuscript in progress at the Brookings
     Institution. See also Patricia Bauman, "The Formulation
     and Evolution of the Health Maintenance Organization
     Policy, 1970-73," Social Science and Medicine, vol. 10
     (1976): 129-42.

(15) Paul M. Ellwood, Jr., et al., "Health Maintenance Strategy," Medical Care, vol. 9 (May-June 1971), pp. 291-98.

(16) Message from the President of the United States Relative to Building a National Health Strategy, House Document No. 92-49, 92 Cong. 1 sess., February 18, 1971, pp. 3-7.

(17) For an historical overview which captures the flavor of this "movement," see William A. MacColl, Group Practice and Prepayment of Medical Care (Washington: Public Affairs Press, 1966).

(18) Group Health Association of America, Inc., Group Health News, vol. 20 (February 1979), p. 1.

(19) This section draws upon the author's research at the Brookings Institution on the politics of health-care regulation. The project is supported by Grant number HS 02932 from the National Center for Health Services Research, OASH.

(20) An example is now-retired Senator Wallace Bennett (R-Utah), a leader of the Senate effort to create PSROs. See John K. Iglehart, "Congress Will Modify Health Programs, Delaying Debate on Broader Reforms," National Journal, February 26, 1972, pp. 365-366.

(21) The proposal is explained and analyzed in detail in William L. Dunn and Bonnie Lefkowitz, "The Hospital Cost Containment Act of 1977: An Analysis of the Administration's Proposal," in Michaele Zubkoff et al. (eds.), Hospital Cost Containment (New York: PRODIST, 1978), pp. 166-214.

(22) The Congressional Budget Office has been looking into the matter, however, and the finance committees in the 96th Congress may well hold hearings on changes in the tax treatment of medical expenditures and health insurance premiums.

(23) On July 18, 1978, the Health Subcommittee of the House Interstate and Foreign Commerce Committee voted by a one-vote margin not to report a revised version of the Carter proposal. In October, however, the Senate surprised observers, including hospital and medical industry lobbyists fighting the bill, by voting 64-22 to attach a cost containment measure to a minor tariff bill. See Congressional Quarterly Weekly Reports, July 22, 1978, pp. 1885-1887, and National Journal, October 21, 1978, p. 1687. Early in the 96th Congress, House Speaker Thomas P. O'Neill predicted that a hospital cost-containment measure "will pass if it gets to the floor," but also surmised that there would be a battle within the closely divided health subcommittee. Dennis Farney, "O'Neill to Fight for Social Programs, Despite Pressures

for Budget-Cutting," The Wall Street Journal, February 5, 1979. About a month later, Carter submitted a new revised hospital cost-containment plan amidst congressional predictions that "the mood is different this year ... and the bill has at least a fighting chance." Victor Cohn, "President Renews His Fight for Hospital Cost Controls," Washington Post, March 7, 1979.

(24) For an excellent discussion of European arrangements, see William A. Glaser, Health Insurance Bargaining: Foreign Lessons for Americans (New York: Gardner Press, 1978).

16 Social Planning and Citizens' Participation: A Discussion and Empirical Analysis, with Data Drawn from the Health Planning Area*

Virginia Cohn Parkum

PARTICIPATION AND PLANNING

Citizen participation in the political system has long been an area of interest to political and social scientists. Whether the "consent of the governed" is obtained through passive acquiescense, as exemplified by the conduct of Bertolt Brecht's Herr Egge,(1) or by varying degrees of activity, beginning with Schumpeter's "free competition among would-be leaders for the vote of the electorate,"(2) is a crucial theoretical and practical issue. It would seem that even the word democracy must be used with asterisks and footnotes for, as Ithiel de Solo Pool notes, there has been a trend in the press toward an increasingly participatory conception of democracy.(3) One person's democracy may be another's prison. The practical implications are reflected in the stresses put on the political system by the advocation of increased citizen participation by various segments of the population.

Indeed, much of the literature advocating increased citizen participation stresses that participation in the traditional sense is ineffective for obtaining the goals of individuals or local communities, for the forms of government

*This study was funded in part by a grant from the Health Services and Mental Health Administration, United States Department of Health, Education, and Welfare, under Section 314(a) of the Public Health Service Act. Additional support was given by the Gesellschaft der Freunde der Universitaet Mannheim for the development of a comparative perspective and the health-planning system efficacy measures.

and political procedures developed under the social and legal
conditions of the eighteenth and nineteenth centuries are
regarded as out-dated for the urbanized, industrialized,
heterogeneous population of today. In 1969, John D. Carroll
discussed what he sensed was a general withering away of
public confidence in the state as an open political order for
structuring such processes as persuasion and bargaining to
make legitimate decisions concerning basic social conflicts.(4)
Carroll felt that planning bodies must accommodate their
awareness of this trend by means of lateral and collegial,
rather than hierarchical, definitions of reality. Donald Haider
cites a number of studies indicating that supporters of urban
reform may be placing too much emphasis on elections as an
essential procedure for ensuring participation and
accountability, affecting policy choices, and increasing the
legitimacy of urban political systems.(5)

The problems of public participation in the reallocation of
resources (values) are reflected in the specific area of
health-policy planning. The need for resource redistribution
is evident, given that everyone has a right to good health and
the health services necessary to provide it. That everyone
has such a right is especially clear in light of the frequently
acknowledged interdependence of individuals today, which
arises in part from the financial inability of many to care
adequately for their health problems.(6) In the United States,
an extensive effort has been made to develop channels for
input by citizens to the health care planning processes.

CHP: A LEGISLATIVE RESPONSE

The Comprehensive Health Planning legislation was part of the
Great Society policy that provided for various forms of
citizens' participation, though it was not generally well known.
The emphasis on consumers' participation represents the
confluence of several trends: consumerism itself;(7) the call
by minority groups and many other citizens for participatory
democracy; the activism of the Civil Rights movement; an
emphasis on decentralizing administration; a wave of
antiprofessionalism and a growing awareness among health and
other professionals of the value of planning services with the
help of the proposed recipients of the service;(8) and the
recognition, often stressed by the news media, that many
health needs were not being met.

Comprehensive Health Planning was created by federal
legislation enacted in November 1966 as Public Law 89-749, the
Comprehensive Health Planning and Public Health Services
Amendments, and by the passage in 1967 of Public Law 90-174,
the Partnership for Health Amendments. The legislation

defined good health in terms of the national interest by stating that "the fulfillment of our national purpose depends on promoting and assuring the highest level of health attainable for every person," thus giving some substance to the purposefully vague reference to welfare in the Constitution.

Basically, each state was formally to designate or establish a specific agency for comprehensive health planning. A council made up of both health consumers and health providers was selected to advise the State Comprehensive Health Planning (CHP) agency. Formula block grants were made to the states on the bases of population and per capita income and were to be spent according to the state CHP proposals, thus replacing the prior system of allocating funds in such federally designated categories as cancer, chronic illness, and dental health.

The state agency was to approve areawide CHP councils or agencies, each of which was to provide comprehensive plans for the more local geographic units it covered. Again, both consumers and providers were to be represented. In contrast, many of the formula health planning efforts in West Germany do not bring citizen/consumer representatives (however they are defined) and providers together in one group until the highest levels of discussion are reached, and not always then. The American states' definitions of "area" in areawide were often based on previously established political jurisdictions that for various reasons had in the past been considered as administrative areas. Thus, the definition of the CHP planning units was not necessarily based on the range of social, political, and economic factors relevant to health and health care.

REGULATIONS ON PARTICIPATION

All Americans are potential consumers of health care, but there was confusion about participation in Comprehensive Health Planning because the concept of consumer was not clearly defined in the law.(9) The areawide agencies and their various committees must "provide for representation of the major public and voluntary agencies, organizations, and institutions concerned with physical, mental, and environmental health services, facilities, and manpower" and "the majority of the membership of the board of directors or advisory council must be consumers of health services broadly reflecting geographic, socioeconomic and ethnic groups in the area." No person whose major occupation is the administration of health activities or performance of health services shall be considered a consumer representative. This requirement also excludes as consumers all persons engaged in research or teaching in

health fields.(10)   Pennsylvania guidelines also stressed that
consumer membership must provide "balanced representation of
the traditionally influential and previously unheard."(11)   It
was   the   responsibility   of   the   areawide   agency   and   its
subgroups to define further the concepts of consumer and
balance for their areas.   No clear formula was given for
establishing either what Paul Peterson has labeled "socially
descriptive representation," measured by the extent to which
representatives accurately reflect the social characteristics of
those whom they formally represent, or Hanna Pitkin's concept
of   "descriptive   representation,"   which   is   measured   by   the
degree to which representatives share the political opinions as
well   as   socioeconomic   status   characteristics   of   their
constituencies.(12)
        The problem of defining who was to be given the op-
portunity to participate was not unique to the CHP legislation.   John Strange notes the various meanings of citizen
which have developed in the experiences of the Office of
Economic   Opportunity   (OEO)   and   the   Model   Cities   programs.(13)   Indeed, determining whose demands should be
turned   into   policies,   or   defining   long-,   middle-,   and
short-term priorities for consuming the limited resources in the
most efficient and effective way without losing support for the
political structure itself, is a systemic problem of governments
today.   In West Germany, trade unions and other formally
organized   occupation-related   organizations   are   generally
accepted in legislation as the carriers of citizen interest.   This
can be seen, for example, in the "social elections" and the
Concerted Action (Konzertierte Aktion) planning bodies.(14)
A similar situation exists de facto in many structures in which
American citizens participate.

DUTIES AND POWERS

The plans developed by the areawide and state units were to
deal with physical, mental, and environmental health needs, as
well as the necessity of the facilities, services, and manpower
required to meet these needs.   Public, voluntary, and private
resources were to be developed and coordinated.   Task forces
and committees were generally formed at local, areawide, and
state levels to focus on each problem.   Some limited say about
resource allocation was provided for through the establishment
of   approval/disapproval   powers   over   certain   plans.(15)
However, the committees had little real power, for the plans
were not binding.

POSTSCRIPT: CHP AFTER
THE COMPLETION OF THE STUDY

Comprehensive Health Planning was seen by some as a major
means for making state and local government programs more
responsive to real needs.(16)   It was to be an exercise in
"creative federalism," shifting program responsibility away
from Washington(17) rather than imposing a master plan by the
federal government upon the people.(18)   Joseph Zimmerman
characterized such policies as attempts to overcome
"politicosclerosis," or hardening of the arteries of political
communication.(19)

However, CHP became neither a widely effective agent of
change, nor a catalyst for restructuring the health services
delivery system, nor a force for organizing a new system for
the promotion of well-being. It was designed to fail in these
respects, inasmuch as the law itself forbids "interference with
existing patterns of private professional practice of medicine,
dentistry, and related arts."

Recent legislation has prescribed the demise of CHP as
such, but it has maintained the goal of comprehensive health
planning, as have measures to provide actual services.   The
National Health Planning and Resources Development Act of
1974 (P.L. 93-641) strengthened the federal government's
commitment to promoting the development of a health-systems
plan from the community level (Health Systems Agencies) on
up, with the eventual achievement of equal access to quality
health care at a reasonable cost mentioned as a federal
government priority.   The key concepts of planning and
development were linked.

The changes, in comparison with the CHP legislation,
seem incremental rather than revolutionary.   The idea of
consumer participation in planning has been retained, and the
scope of consumer influence has been potentially broadened by
the increase of the resource allocation power of the Health
Systems Agencies. The mere use of the word "systems" does
not automatically assure the systematization of the planning
and control of the $85 billion health provision and services
industry, but the new organizational framework may be a step
in that direction if the consumer and provider members are so
inclined.

CONSUMERS MEET PROVIDERS:
A STUDY OF CHP COMMITTEES

The study reported here was an attempt to evaluate the
correctness of the assumptions made in the legislation about

the operational components of the program structure, which in this case are the members of the community health planning committees. The assumptions concern the attitudes hypothetically held by the members and the actions these attitudes are presumed to foster.

The attitudinal "fit" is potentially crucial to the functioning of the entire program as envisioned by its designers. The program structure was based on implicit or explicit assumptions about the relationship between attitudes and behavior of the various types of committee members, and the setting of health consumer/health provider was seen as one of both cooperation and conflict. That the assumptions sometimes ran contrary to various social science theories made the evaluation all the more interesting.

An extension of the concept of political efficacy was used in examining how the committee members felt about their influence regarding general community health decision-making (external health-system efficacy) and their influence in the specific planning committees (internal health-planning system efficacy).

The study examines a sample of the community-health planning committee membership in three demographically different areas in Pennsylvania. The total sample size was 210 - 98 health consumers and 112 providers. Two sets of interviews were conducted; they were separated by a year so that change over time could be studied. Meetings of various units were observed during the same period. This is one of few studies on citizens' participation in community-planning organizations based on a sample selected according to scientific procedures.(20)

Given the legislative mandate, the public desires of various interested groups, and the actual community environment, who in fact became members of CHP committee? Almost half the sample were managers, administrators, proprietors, or officials. About 40 percent of the consumers fell into these categories, as did 50 percent of the providers. Almost all the providers and, more remarkably, about 21 percent of the consumers, felt they had health-related occupations.

Most of the respondents were from the middle or upper class and were reasonably well-off economically. Many voluntary community-planning organizations in the United States share this characteristic, as do most of the citizen-action groups in the Federal Republic of Germany.(21)

A large majority of the respondents were between 40 and 59 years old, and nearly half were women. A majority of both consumers and providers were college graduates. Eighty-six percent of the consumers were white, as were almost all of the providers.

Experience in committee work was far from lacking. Most members, regardless of category, were quite active in numerous other associations.

The distribution according to political affiliation was fairly even among Democrats, Republicans, and independents, with no significant difference between consumers and providers. However, a number of respondents, though not a majority, believed that most providers were Republicans and most consumers were Democrats.

People said that they volunteered for the Comprehensive Health Planning work primarily for four general reasons: (1) they explained that participation was consistent with their values, which were to improve health and welfare conditions, to do something for the community, and cooperate to meet the needs for planning; (2) they felt they had the abilities required, specifically because of their education, work experience, or community organization experience; (3) they wanted to accomplish certain goals, namely to increase their knowledge and to improve community health services; and (4) they believed that the people who accept involvement habitually accept community responsibilities.

Consumers in particular tended to emphasize the desire to do something for the community, and they also reported joining because they are in the habit of accepting community involvement. Providers emphasized a desire to improve health and welfare conditions, and they also more often pointed out their ability in terms of education and general background.

The beliefs and attitudes of the people who worked in CHP as volunteers were of major importance for their involvement. In general, it was found that the beliefs and attitudes of consumers were very similar to those of the providers, and that for analytical purposes it usually was more useful to divide people into different categories according to their attitudes rather than according to reference categories defined by social and economic characteristics.

Consumers sometimes felt that their beliefs differed from those of providers because of discrepancies in education and because providers were interested in medicine as a business. Providers sometimes expressed the feeling that they were more knowledgeable, educated, or experienced than consumers and that they were more objective. Yet most in both categories felt that their beliefs did not differ much from those of the members of the opposing category. Respondents in both categories also had favorable feelings about the involvement of lay people as well as the involvement of health professionals.

A frequently mentioned reason for involving consumers was that they knew how well health care was being delivered and could best evaluate the health-care system. The reason most often given for involving providers was that they had expertise and knowledge of the community's needs. They were therefore thought to be of most use in providing professional knowledge and in setting priorities.

Most people agreed with the way consumer participation was being implemented, and they tended to feel, although not strongly, that planning should be done by local people. They felt that a change in the organization of health services was urgent, particularly at the national level, but also at the local level.

Both providers and consumers usually agreed on the goals for their work in CHP, and for the most part they felt that their effort in CHP attained its goals. They felt that their most important accomplishments were in the area of organization; this area was also where they had their most difficult problems.

Most respondents believed that they were given an opportunity to express their points of view in the organization and that their attendance at committee meetings was important. Most reported taking part in committee discussions every time or almost every time.

The work done by most respondents, both consumers and providers, consisted of reviewing and commenting on proposals, participating in discussions, and organizing activities. A large majority came to the committee meetings regularly and spent a few hours or less each month on Comprehensive Health Planning work. Most met between formal meetings to talk over committee affairs with other members.

The amount of time required for involvement was the greatest personal handicap to both consumers and providers in their CHP work. Over half the members had to travel a distance of thirteen or more miles to the meetings. Consumers also often felt hindered by a lack of knowledge about health. The respondents believed these problems also affected other CHP members.

Despite the potential for conflicts, the meeting atmosphere was predominantly friendly. Consumers and providers seldom had radically different ideas about health planning and related topics. Proposal, review, or study problems and problems of committee or council structure were the topics frequently discussed. Disagreements most often occurred when specific health issues and the programs they would necessitate were considered. Disagreements were generally settled by extensive discussion and majority vote. The lively confrontations that many theorists and organized health interests feared and that some participation advocates hoped for seldom occurred in these committees. Also, while there were relatively few differences between the general attitudes of consumers and providers, the providers tended to become increasingly more involved than the consumers, which was the very thing CHP's designers hoped to prevent.

A majority of both health consumers and providers had high feelings of efficacy within the CHP committee and mixed feelings about their effectiveness in dealing with problems in the health-care "system" in general. Very few differences were found between consumer and provider responses when controlled for income, race, age, sex, and education. Respondents 60 years old or older were more inclined than the rest of the members to feel they did not have much say in the committee decisions. The middle-age respondents replied more often than the younger or older members that they had a great or very great say. Regarding the respondents' understanding of health planning issues facing their communities, the providers tended to express stronger feelings of understanding than did the consumers, and, interestingly enough in light of the rhetoric calling for the poor to be active in planning, a comparatively large percentage of the low-income participants, both consumers and providers, felt they had little understanding of the issues. As a group, the black respondents tended to be somewhat more action-oriented than the white members; most of them (about 97 percent) who responded to the question felt they would try to a great or very great extent to change a harmful health regulation, whereas only about 77 percent of the whites felt that way. It should be emphasized that little support overall was shown for the hypothesis that providers have a stronger sense of efficacy.

That strong feelings of efficacy within the committee at one point will be related to high degrees of participation at a later point has a rather firm backing, derived from other studies. Regarding CHP committee work, a higher sense of internal efficacy at the time of the first interview was positively related to a high degree of participation after one year, despite the low resource-allocation power involved in CHP decisions.

CONCLUSION

If participatory democracy is seen as seeking to create structures that involve people in decisions that affect their lives, then CHP embodied this general orientation. However, actual participation in CHP committees reflects the pluralist view, abhorred by many advocates of participatory democracy, of a relatively limited number of consistently active members continually participating and demanding resources of the system. Given both the theory that justifies and inspires participation and the opportunity, in the form of an issue-related organization, to become active, people do not necessarily find participation desirable.

Nevertheless, planning committees involving community participation are another type of formal linkage between the public and policy. They give some muscles to the skeletal macroframework Amitai Etzioni built in his active society.(22) They are not units of "primary democracy"(23) in which all citizens affected by the decisions which the committees make or administer may always participate directly, but rather are elements of some form of representative government in which only selected community members hold positions. However, this representative organ is closer physically to the citizen's community than the federal or state government, and it deals more directly with decisions involving specific issues such as health planning than the local citizen's elected representatives in city, state, or national governments often do.

Such participation of citizens in the planning process can produce plans that are acceptable to experts and are also acceptable to the affected populations, because of their more direct involvement in the planning process itself. This process embodies the problems of consensus and consent which have occupied generations of political scientists and theorists. Carefully applied citizen's participation may be a partial solution to the malaise and lack of confidence in governmental institutions said to be affecting the postindustrial, postwelfare societies.(24) True, "The best laid scheme o' mice and men/Gang aft a-gley."(25) But with a planning process designed to consider programs in light of the limited resources, needs, and desires of specific populations, it seems that the chances for making useful plans that are accepted by the public as legitimate and for having them enacted as intended should be increased.

NOTES

(1) For seven years Herr Egge served an agent of the authorities who was quartered in his home. He carried out all actions demanded of him but never answered the question "Will you serve me?" until after the official was dead and buried, at which time Herr Egge breathed a sigh of relief and replied "No." From Bertolt Brecht, "Massnahmen gegen die Gewalt," Geschichten vom Herrn Keuner (Frankfurt/M: Suhrkamp, 1972), pp. 9-10.
(2) Joseph A. Schumpeter, Capitalism, Socialism, and Democracy, 3d ed. (New York: Harper and Row, Harper Torchbooks, 1950).
(3) Ithiel de Solo Pool, The Prestige Press: A Comparative Study of Political Symbols (Cambridge, Mass.: M.I.T. Press, 1970), pp. 194-218.

(4)   John D. Carroll, "Noetic Authority," Public Administra-
      tion Review, 29 (September-October) 1969, pp. 492-500.
(5)   Donald Haider, "The Political Economy of Decentraliza-
      tion," American Behavioral Scientist, 15:1 (September/Oc-
      tober) 1971, 108-129.
(6)   For a detailed discussion see Virginia Cohn Parkum,
      Efficacy and Action, dissertation, University of Mannheim,
      West Germany, 1976, pp. 9-40.
(7)   This is sometimes labeled the "consumer offensive," as
      on ABC-TV, "The Consumer Offensive - Who Speaks for
      the People?" November 29, 1975, which reviewed the
      growth of the consumer movement in the sixties and its
      implications today. For analyses of the movement see
      Alan Gartner and Frank Riessman, The Service Society
      and the Consumer (New York: Harper & Row, 1974) and
      Mark V. Nadel, "Consumerism: A Coalition in Flux,"
      Policy Studies Journal, 4:1 (Autumn 1975), pp. 31-35.
(8)   The acceptance and advocacy of this latter viewpoint
      today at the international level can be seen in United
      Nations, Economic and Social Council, Commission for
      Social Development, 24th Session, Popular Participation
      and Its Practical Implications for Development: Notes by
      the Secretary-General (E/CN.5/496), 15 August 1974.
(9)   Lawrence F. Bennett, "The Role of Dentistry in
      Federal-State-Local Comprehensive Health Planning,"
      Journal of Public Health Dentistry 28 (Fall), 1968, p.
      218; Boyd Z. Palmer et al., "Community Participation in
      the Planning Process," Health Education Monographs 32
      (1972), p. 6.
(10) U.S. Department of Health, Education, and Welfare,
      Public Health Service, Office of Comprehensive Health
      Planning, "Information and Policies on Grants for Com-
      prehensive Areawide Health Planning. Section 314 (b),
      Public Health Service Act as amended by PL 89-749."
      Washington, D.C. (August 30, 1967), p. 6.
(11) Pennsylvania Department of Health, Office of Com-
      prehensive Health Planning, Guidelines for Consumer
      Representation on Areawide Comprehensive Health
      Planning Agencies, p. 2.
(12) Paul E. Peterson, "Forms of Representation: Participation
      of the Poor in the Community Action Program," American
      Political Science Review 64:2 (June) 1970, 492; Hanna
      Pitkin, The Concept of Representation (Berkeley: Univer-
      sity of California Press, 1967), especially Chapter 4.
(13) John H. Strange, "The Impact of Citizen Participation on
      Public Administration," PAR 32 (September) 1972, pp.
      459-460.
(14) These are discussed by Henry A. Landsberger in "The
      Trend toward 'Citizen Participation' in the Welfare State:
      Countervailing Power to the Professions?" Paper pre-

sented at the 9th World Congress of Sociology (Workshop
10), Uppsala, Sweden, August 14-19, 1978; and Cost-
Control in the Federal Republic of Germany: Lessons for
the United States? U.S. Department of Health, Education
and Welfare, National Center for Health Information
(forthcoming).

(15) Robert M. Corbett, "Health Planning - Some Legal and
Political Implications of Comprehensive Health Planning,"
American Journal of Public Health 64:2 (February 1974),
pp. 136-139. Corbett discusses CHP's review areas.

(16) Eugene Guthrie, "The Potential of Planning," Bulletin of
the New York Academy of Medicine 44 (February 1968),
pp. 113-119.

(17) Douglas Cater, "Community Health Planning: Creative
Federalism," American Journal of Public Health 58 (June
1968), p. 1024.

(18) W. H. Stewart, "Comprehensive Health Planning." Ad-
dress to the National Health Forum of the National Health
Council, Chicago, March 21, p. 11, quoted in Lewis D.
Polk, "The Comprehensive Health Planning Laws from the
Local Viewpoint," Public Health Reports 84 (January
1969), p. 90.

(19) Joseph F. Zimmerman, "Neighborhoods and Citizen Involvement," PAR 32:3 (May/June 1972), p. 209.

(20) For an extensive presentation of the basic data derived
from the study, see Kurt H. Parkum and Virginia C.
Parkum, Voluntary Participation in Health Planning, Har-
risburg, Pennsylvania: Pennsylvania Department of
Health, 1973.

(21) See Kurt H. Parkum and Virginia C. Parkum, "Citizen
Participation in Planning and Decision-Making: Shaping
the Community," in David Horton Smith and Jacqueline
Macaulay, eds., Informal Social Participation (San
Francisco: Jossey-Bass, forthcoming). Bruce C. Vladeck
discusses this problem in the HSA's, CHP's successor
bodies, in "Interest-Group Representation and the
HSA's," AJPH 67:1 (January 1977), pp. 23-29. The
Urban Studies Institute in West Berlin released the
German figures.

(22) Amitai Etzioni, The Active Society (New York: The Free
Press), 1968. At Etzioni's request, Warren Breed wrote a
shorter version of the book, which was published as The
Self-Guiding Society (New York: The Free Press, 1971),
p. 152.

(23) Robert Dahl, After The Revolution? (New Haven: Yale
University Press, 1970).

(24) See also Max Kaase, "Political Ideology and Political Participation: New Pressures on Old Institutions?", paper, Colloquium on Overloaded Government, Florence, December 13-17, 1976.

(25) Robert Burns, "To a Mouse," stanza 7.

17 The Trend Toward Citizens' Participation in the Welfare State: Countervailing Power to the Professions

Henry A. Landsberger

This paper proposes a thesis which is unusual and, given the mood of the times, may even be unpopular. The typical posture today on both the left and the right is one of pessimism about the political systems of the neocapitalist democracies. In those who tend toward the left, their pessimism is adorned with just a little Schadenfreude; in those who tend toward the right, there is a note of subdued alarm. In either case, the prevalent image is one of a possible rupture of the existing system in the not too distant future.

The thesis here, by way of contrast, is - at least mildly - positive and optimistic. It affirms that visible and effective effort, in varying but, on the whole, considerable quantities, has been made in the last ten or fifteen years in the expanding neocapitalist welfare states of the North Atlantic to broaden, establish, and extend new institutionalized forms of citizen participation. There are interesting differences among states in the manner in which these provisions for participation are structured, in the extent to which they exist at all; and in the speed with which they have expanded. Our thesis is that differences in the manner in which different countries have structured citizen's participation are indicative of inherently and unavoidably difficult choices between certain principles which underlie the concept of citizen's participation. The conflict of these principles is inevitable; they represent genuine dilemmas. No structure of participation can ever be totally satisfactory.

LITERATURE

Some elaboration is necessary to fit this thesis into the contemporary discussion of participation and the supposed malaise of the democratic state. In the United States, research has focused, as is customary there, on the relevant political attitudes and behaviors of the individual and their correlates. In the academic world, this line of research is best represented by the work of Milbrath (1964, 1974) as well as by that of Almond and Verba (1965) and Verba and Nie (1973). In the world of practical politics, the current pessimism is to some extent justified in the United States by declining voter participation in elections and by public opinion polls which indicate declining confidence in the major political institutions of the United States and especially in its elected representatives.

In addition to these empirical studies at the level of the individual, there are also mildly critical and pessimistic system-oriented discussions concerning the relationship between democracy and participation (Bachrach, 1970; Bachrach and Baratz, 1970). Above all, there is unease about the normative significance and the practical consequences of the kind of pluralistic elitism which seems to characterize the American political system. It appears that various elites compete and negotiate with each other under only the very remote and sporadic supervision of the voter, who may merely legitimate the process rather than genuinely control it. Yet, on the right, in the United States as in Europe, there is fear that increased participation would result in excess demand on the state. On the left, there is the prediction that a merely formal, substantively sham democracy cannot and ought not to last.

This kind of fundamental criticism of the existing political structure is much more systematic and comprehensive in the political science literature of Germany. It certainly occupies there a proportionately larger place, perhaps only because the mass of empirical studies of attitudes and voting that characterizes political science writings in the United States does not exist to a comparable extent in Germany. Concepts such as verwaltungsstaat (the administrative state), burgerfremde (estrangement of the state from the citizen) - terms which merge concept, description, and normative rejection - flourish in the literature. This can be seen in the very thorough summary by Aleman and his collaborators (Aleman, 1978).

This reader's unease with that literature, which is balanced by similar unease with much of the directionless empiricism in the United States, stems from the lack of substantial data to support claims about the supposed crisis of the system, which is either stated to exist already or is forecast to be more or less imminent. These claims appear to be as much reflections of the authors' own norms and images about what a real democracy should be as they are empirically grounded assessments. The reader never quite knows to what extent an author is predicting a breakdown on the basis of well analyzed facts or a prophetic gloom that arises from a feeling that a system as bad as this must and should suffer some kind of purging, since the world is ultimately just. Authors on the right, such as Hennis (1973), also speculate about a day of reckoning, which they believe will come because the idea of democracy has been extended conceptually, practically, and normatively in ways that it cannot and ought not to be. This reader has found the literature, although it is extraordinarily stimulating, to blend in an often confusing manner the supposedly conceptual, the strictly factual, and the personal, normative, and ideological.

There has not been in Germany a notable decline in voter participation nor a notable increase in voter alienation from the parties. Yet these facts are rarely mentioned! It is true that the last 15 years have seen the birth and growth of extraparliamentary citizens' initiatives (Burgerinitiativen) and, recently, their move into politics through the "green" and "multicolored" lists. Since these spontaneous citizens' protests could be interpreted as heralding the hoped for (or the feared) apocalypse, they have indeed been studied. (For summaries, see Mayer-Tasch, 1977; and Armbruster and Leisner, 1975).

Despite what the literature may indicate, logic dictates that calamity is not around the corner. This seems especially clear when one compares these recent, mild demands for participation (made in the ante-room of parliamentary politics, as German political scientists call it) with the kind of mass unrest which in the past has preceded major political changes; the unrest in Germany between the two World Wars is a convenient example. In any case, and central to this paper: It is intriguing and relatively overlooked that governments have created or have expanded many new institutions to enable citizens to participate more continuously and broadly in the myriad decisions that an expanding welfare state necessarily makes. (The traditional method of participation is, of course, the election of representatives to national, regional and communal governments which supposedly do, but in practice cannot, supervise all the multitude of services offered by the state. Very occasionally, there are referenda and plebiscites on an inevitably limited number of issues). Whether the new mechanisms of participation which we describe below are intended to be merely ways of legitimizing and stabilizing regimes, and whether they actually have that effect or some other effect, is a logical next question. But that question

cannot even be asked until the phenomenon of the growth of
new participatory institutions is recognized.

NEW INSTITUTIONALIZED FORMS OF PARTICIPATION

In the United States of America, "maximum feasible participation" made a dramatic debut in 1964 as part of the War on
Poverty (Economic Opportunity Act, Section 201). From the
Boards of Community Action Agencies, the principle spread
rapidly to education (parent advisory committees are mandatory
in Title I programs of the Elementary and Secondary Education
Act of 1965); to the Boards of Neighborhood Health Centers
and Community Mental Health Centers; to Model Cities and,
most recently, to the entire area of national health planning.
The Natoinal Health Planning and Resource Development Act of
1974 (PL 93-641) makes mandatory that there be a 'consumer'
majority on the governing boards of the 210 newly created
Health Systems Agencies (HSA's) which now cover the United
States.
          In the United Kingdom, Community Health Councils have
been put astride the three administrative layers of the National
Health Service (Regional and Area Health Authorities, and
District Management Teams) to serve a very active 'watch-dog'
function. The just-published (August 1979) report of the
Royal Commission on the National Health Service assesses their
effectiveness very positively, and recommends that their
functions and powers be extended. In the field of urban
planning and renewal, the so-called Skeffington Report,
"People and Planning," issued in 1969, recommended increased
participation in planning by the public, and the 1971 Town and
Country Planning Act and subsequent Circulars from the
Department of the Department of the Environment have
implemented these recommendations. An increased role for
parents and various community groups (labour, management,
churches) in the management of schools was proposed in
September 1978 by the Taylor Committee in its report, titled
significantly: "A New Partnership for our Schools."
          In the Federal Republic of Germany, legislation and
practice at the state level have steadily enlarged the role
played by parents either through voluntary parents' associations (Elternvereine) and/or through statutorily established parents' advisory councils (Elternbeiraete) and their
participation in higher-level councils, i.e., at the level
of the city or district, the "Land" (state), and the Federal
Republic. In the state of North Rhine Westphalia (Germany's
most populous state) such parent organizations, in conjunction
with some of the teacher unions and supported also by the
opposition Christian Democratic Union, successfully sponsored

a 'petition' to the parliament of that state which led it to rescind an already approved law giving local authorities permission to establish 'comprehensive' secondary schools on an experimental basis. A modest enough proposal, but enough to successfully arouse these parents. In the field of urban planning, various revisions of the federal statutes governing urban construction and renewal since 1969 have made consultation with affected citizens increasingly more formalized and mandated. And in the field of health, the entire system is designed to provide for 'bargaining' between providers and sickness funds, in the latter of which employers and trade unions (on behalf of worker-contributors) hold equal power. The trade unions, understandably, have a greater interest in the system, and seek to pursue through it well-formulated and innovative health policies. The system has existed for almost one hundred years, and recent legislation enhances the power of the Sickness Funds vis a vis providers (physicians' associations and hospitals) and hence the power of consumers.

It is our thesis, however, that desirable though these attempts to given citizens more power may be, they necessarily confront certain dilemmas of structure and policy; it is to these that we now turn.

FOUR STRUCTURAL PROBLEMS

There is a temptation to think that the "reproductive" social service state deals with ("exploits"?) a fairly unified, homogeneous body of citizens. This temptation is not altogether dissimilar from the assumption made in the past that there is a homogeneous, potentially united, and exploited working class or that there would be such a class once the workers became fully aware of their condition and shed their false consciousness.

Very early in the evolution of ideas about the restructuring of the productive sector, when ideas were formulated about changing the relationship of labor to capital, it became clear that "the enemy," capital, could be located with some ease. (Even doing that seems much more difficult now we know, as Marx suspected, that a state bureaucracy might easily take the place of private capital.) But right from the beginning, there were obvious problems in defining "the hero," at least once a priori assumptions and generalities were left behind. For example, to leave power in the hands of the workers of a particular plant, or even of a particular industry (workers who were themselves probably neither homogeneous nor of one mind) was considered by most to be inequitable. For that reason, Syndicalism was not widely supported: because it ignored "the general good" and left out the consumer, a danger of which GDH and Margaret Cole warned even in their "guild socialism" phase. Recent discussions have not, of course, produced either a clear-cut conceptual solution or a practical solution to this insoluble issue. (See the summaries of various recent positions in Ehrhardt, et al., pp. 112 passim, in Alemann, 1978.)

In the "reproductive" social service state, as in the productive sector there are really four different but related issues which are parallel to the historical one we have just described. The first problem is who exactly the "public" is. Is it homogeneous, or are there many and various constituencies whose interests may be as opposed to those of the others as they are to those of the "providers" of social services? For example, do the younger contributors to pension funds perceive their interests to be very different from those of older contributors? If such is the case, then how can one delimit these constituencies according to any principle of legitimacy? How and by whom and according to what principles are they actually delimited? A more fundamental question is: if "citizens" can be seen as merely another set of special-interest groups, are they so fundamentally different from others, i.e., from providers? What principle of legitimacy justifies conceding more power to them than to other actors?

A somewhat similar problem arises on the other side. Those advocating citizen participation usually perceive the "enemy" of the citizen to be the professions that provide services, such as physicians, teachers, planners, social workers, and the administering state. This view parallels the way that the bourgeoisie, politicians, and bureaucrats were and, in part, still are conceptualized in the classic Marxist picture of exploitation in the productive sector.

But how united, for that matter, are the providers? In Germany recently, during negotiations over a new Health Cost Control Law, physicians sacrificed the interests of the pharmaceutical industry without too much hesitation. And within the health profession, there are tensions between hospital physicians and those in private practice. Are the interests of providers necessarily so much narrower and more self-serving than those of limited groups of citizens if the latter are viewed soberly and are not romanticized? And if the professionals are not really quite as uniquely arbitrary and antisocial in the exercise of their power as they may seem to be, is the power they wield as professionals really quite so lacking in legitimacy as is sometimes claimed?

The point here is that groups of citizens and providers consist of a large number of actors all of whom are selfish to a degree which is substantial, even if it may be difficult to assess. Because of this difficulty, both analysts and the state have trouble determining both how bad the present situation is and by how much it would really be improved by reallocating power.

The second problem facing those who wish to institutionalize citizens' participation in the social services is determining how new participants should participate. Should they do so in an unmediated fashion, through direct democracy, or should they do so through an interest organization? The latter possibility raises the specter, once again, of an unrepresentative and insensitive oligarchy and bureaucracy, such as those that control some trade unions. Yet without organization (as in the case of America's Health System Agencies) citizens, however they are defined, are likely to be ineffectual and weak. They cannot devote themselves full-time to participation, and they lack adequate knowledge to participate in fields that are highly technical. Participation in policy formation at the national level is practically impossible without representation through organizations. Yet there are serious drawbacks to participation through interest organizations.

The third problem is determining how participation should be structured. Should the citizens or consumers be integrated into the decision-making structure essentially in a Mitbestimmung pattern, through codetermination? Or should they remain independent outsiders? If they should remain outside the decision process, in what posture should they do so? Should they be critics (as in England's CHC's) or should they be bargainers? On the one hand, only by being inside can they share in ongoing decision making and, above all, influence administrative policy, which is so important in the welfare sectors. But the danger in that case is that they will be overwhelmed or co-opted by the greater status and technical expertise of their codeciders. Remaining outside would assure them independence, but it almost certainly would limit the amount of information available to them for formulating alternative policies and criticisms.

The fourth problem is determining the relationship of new participatory institutions to pre-existing parliamentary structures, especially local ones. These popularly elected local bodies are supposed to represent the local citizen already. Moreover, local and higher levels of government (counties, states, Lander) usually have standing committees to consider policy matters in the spheres of health, education, and city planning, to supervise the respective administrative bureaucracies, and to deal with special interests and lobbies. These government structures were intended to be adequate to represent the citizen.

It is clear that in some countries at least, local and central governments and elected representatives are in bad repute at the moment, even though academics may well be

exaggerating the extent and the significance of public dissatisfaction with them. However, the establishment, through
legislation, of new mechanisms that enable citizens to participate, indicates that legislatures have themselves accepted
implicitly or explicitly the contemporary criticism of the
adequacy of popular representation through the existing array
of institutions.

But however much their legitimacy as representatives
may have been compromised, local elected officials do in fact
have power, including the power to protect their power. And
even their claim to be legitimately representative may not be so
unjust on a comparative basis. They claim, perhaps accurately, that they are elected by more people, in a more
open process, than any of the individuals in the new, rival
participation structures. Will the new structures be, and
appear to be, so much more 'legitimate' than the old?

NEW PARTICIPATION IN URBAN PLANNING,
HEALTH, AND EDUCATION: HOW IT FUNCTIONS

Urban planning. In the United Kingdom, the Federal Republic
of Germany and the United States, it is clearly the traditional
local and regional authorities who make the final decisions in
the area of urban planning. Provisions to increase the
participation of citizens who are most directly affected by
urban plans have been made, but they do not in practice
increase that participation by very much. The acknowledgment
of the right to be heard and to comment early is the extent of
the new concessions.

How can this relatively small increase in opportunities for
participation be explained? The increase was politically
necessary because of severe local reactions in all three
countries to having superhighways slice through and destroy
residential areas; to the elimination of old but cheap housing
duirng urban renewal programs and the consequent dis-
placement to inconvenient city peripheries of persons who
could least afford it, and to other such policies. The
intensity of local reaction forced the state to soften somewhat
the manner in which it exercised the authority it ultimately
retained.

But it went no further - first, probably, for the rather
pragmatic reason that there was not enough of a pressing
political reason to do so. In other words, restiveness over
urban planning is not general and continuous, but is rather
sporadic and at any one time confined to the place affected.
In this respect, it is very different from the problem of cost
explosion in the field of health, where the rise in contribution rates can cause unease throughout the nation. Issues

concerning schools and hospitals are present all the time, and parents, contributors and patients are always intensely involved with them. In the case of local urban problems, the only national organizations likely to exist are those of landlords and small shop-keepers, which do exist in Germany. But they are weak in any given locality and are not of much interest to the kind of lawmaker who has pushed legislation to facilitate participation.

As for the degree of new power over urban renewal and highway construction which might be given to the local population (whether organized or not, homogeneous or not) as compared to the existing local authorities, the latter clearly have a good deal of legitimacy on their side. For in many cases, the projects are explicitly undertaken for the benefit of sectors of the population beyond that immediately affected, and it is appreciated that there will be a local "cost." The balancing of all interests, including wider ecological ones, is obviously very difficult. But giving a great deal of power to a limited, local community may not be any more defensible than ignoring it totally.

Thus, the technical difficulties of organizing and of delimiting appropriate interest groups and reasonably plausible arguments of equity would tend to limit local citizen power quite severely, even if mammoth financial interests of all kinds did not do so. And in the capitalist societies of the west, financial interests have obviously and clearly been the beneficiaries of the existing system of local power distribution, which they seek to perpetuate.

Health. The following tentative generalizations can be made about citizen participation in the health field: (1) The new participatory institutions in the health field are stronger and have advanced more dramatically than those in the field of urban planning. The chief explanations are that (a) public dissatisfaction in this field is more general, more persistent, and stronger than in the other, and (b) the governments concerned needed the power of citizens to back up the various policies and measures which they, the governments, wished to adopt. (2) Nevertheless, preexisting institutional structures (such as the German sickness funds and physicians' groups) and power distributions (such as the greater power of local government in Britain) can be modified, but cannot, of course, be overturned, abolished, or ignored in favor of any new structure. (3) In neither urban renewal nor in health is there one unified constituency or even a limited number of self-evidently legitimate constituencies into which citizens can be subdivided. There is no strong esprit de corps among consumers. Hence, it is likely that there will be much divergence among citizens, arising from differences in their interests, backgrounds and values. The chances are that a weak, not very united front will confront the providers. While the latter are in turn not necessarily homogeneous and lacking in conflicts of interest, they are likely to learn to cooperate quickly. (4) Germany and Britain have long kept the citizen outside the main decision-making structure in the field of health. The United States in a way has not done so; at least in the new Health Systems Agencies, personnel intermingle. On the whole, it seems that independence, i.e., the British system of Community Health Councils and the German system of Sickness Funds enables citizens to more successfully defend their points of view.

Education. In the area of education, the relative scarcity of issues that affect more than the individual school or district is one reason why dramatic, area-wide activism is not frequent. (The exception is the issue, in the United Kingdom and Germany, of making secondary education comprehensive, and the issue in the United States of integration.) Furthermore, groups other than parents can be involved, which complicates organization of "the" citizen's faction. These groups include other taxpayers, employers and trade unions. Complicating matters even more is that parents' groups are often divided internally.

Provisions for parental participation tend, for the most part, to keep them separate from the decision making hierarchy and subordinate to the traditional elected authorities. In Britain, the power of local authorities is so substantial and so recognized that even when an expansion of the role of parents is under discussion, as in the 1977 Taylor Report, provision is made to include representatives of local education authorities in the revitalized school-governing bodies. This makes codecision-making bodies similar to the health system agencies in the United States. But whether they are elected boards, as in the United States, or ministries responsible to parliaments, as in Germany, or directors of education responsible to education committees, as in England: it is with traditional bodies that the ultimate authority in education continues to lie.

THE ROLE OF POLITICAL PARTIES

There is one set of established actors outside the new participatory institutions whose relations to these institutions have not yet been discussed. They pose a fifth set of dilemmas. These established actors are the traditional political parties, which present the new participation structures with yet another problem. The parties themselves are naturally enough always eager to attract new members. They are therefore ready to support any new cause which fits in reasonably well with their ideology, provided that it does not offend the more mundane interests of current supporters.* The kinds of substantive issues which arise in the social-service sectors of welfare states frequently lend themselves to being adopted into the program of one party or another. For example, in Britain and Germany, the Labour Parties and the Social Democrats have been identified quite clearly with the movement to establish comprehensive schools. Indeed, the movement was not at all initiated by parents; rather, it came directly from the parties. Their opponents, the British Conservative Party and CDU, respectively, are identified with maintaining the existing tracked system. Hence, parents opposed to the comprehensive school movement are logical recruits for the more conservative parties, which are only too pleased to support them.** As we have already mentioned, the organization of a recent petition in the state of North Rhine Westphalia opposing the Gesamtschule experiment was strongly supported by the CDU. The party is reported to have spent $2.5 million on the campaign, and the support it has gained as a result has been predicted by many as likely to influence subsequent elections.

In the field of health, there is, of course, some tendency for the left to initiate demands for the equalization of access to services and for the regulation of the incomes of doctors and the expenditures of hospitals. This is so because parties of the left are less wedded than others to solving social problems through the market mechanism and are more solicitous of the needs of the less advantaged. In the field of urban renewal the parties of the left are more likely to feel affinity for the the kind of economically deprived portions of the population that are usually most disadvantaged by urban renewal schemes.

However, while the situation may be fairly straightforward for one or other of the established parties, the dilemma for those in the new participatory structures is that they may not wish to become identified with any one party. This is an old dilemma, faced originally by the trade-union movement around the turn of the century. Should

---

*This is the problem faced by the SPD and the Labour Party in connection with environmental issues, especially nuclear power, in their relations with the new ecology groups concerned with policies in these fields. Ideologically, these parties could be environmental protectionists. But their trade-union supporters are on the other side of the fence.

**There are variations. In Niedersachsen (the state of Lower Saxony), it was the CDU which initially introduced Gesamtschulen.

these new participation groups be allied with the parties with which their positions so frequently coincide? Or is there too great a danger that, by becoming associated with one party and antagonizing the other the cause would be damaged when that other party is in power? Many parents, too, although they are against comprehensive schools, do not have any sympathy with Conservatives and the CDU, and would disassociate themselves from the new mechanisms if they became allied with these parties. They also know that if a party in effect takes over an association of parents, as is reputed to have happened in some states in Germany, the state governments will write off the parents' concerns as merely electoral politics. Yet these organizations of parents also do not wish to refuse whatever aid is offered them. The situation is, of course, often much more complex. There are sometimes links between groups and portions of parties. In one city in Germany, a new form of participation in urban renewal planning was tried out only because the left-leaning faction in the SPD in that city got the upper hand at a certain moment. When it lost control, the experiment was discontinued. A further complication is that not only the major parties, but also certain minor groups, especially some on the extreme left, may take an interest in issues of urban renewal, school reform, and so forth, which raises problems for the public images of these new participatory structures.

In any case, political parties are almost certain to be interested in the affairs of new participatory institutions; some regard this situation as a mixed blessing, while others will feel quite comfortable about the involvement of parties. It seems clear, however, that the help of political parties or of sections of them is often crucial to the success of the new institutions; it is certainly crucial to the delineation of the issues. It is the existence of a relatively ideologically coherent party system in Germany and Britain, organizationally strong from center down to the local level, which accounts substantially for the extent to which consumer issues are clearly articulated and ultimately attended to. In the United States, the party system is unable to play the same role. There may well be quite a high price to pay in the long run for having a coherent party system: there may arise a nationwide polarization. There is no such polarization in the United States, and many in both Germany and Britain worry that it may soon arise in their countries. But leaving aside these more general and long-run considerations of the effects of a coherent party system, it seems clear that those issues which can be coordinated with party interests and ideology, as most of them can be, will be taken up by the parties, which at the very least enhances their chances of being clearly debated.

THE FINAL PROBLEM: PARTICIPATION VERSUS MORE
IMPORTANT SOCIAL GOALS INCLUDING
CONTROLLING THE POWER OF THE PROFESSION

There is a sixth and final problem which has not been discussed. The five already discussed are problems involving the inevitable choices which have to be made in structuring a new participatory mechanism. But what if there are "costs" attached to participation in any form that are of such a magnitude that they cast doubt on the worthwhileness of participation itself? The costs referred to here are not the usual opportunity costs of effort and time, which are sufficiently weighty by themselves to raise questions about the viability of new participatory mechanisms. The costs referred to here are potential costs to the public good. What if opening the doors to participation results in the pursuit of popular goals which, from an "objective" point of view, are clearly undesirable for the public welfare? What people want may not be what they ought to want.* As we have seen, parental involvement in the education field is particularly intense and wide-spread, just as one would wish it to be. However, much of this parental enthusiasm has been directed toward preventing the establishment of comprehensive integrated schools, which is not the side on which those advocating "participation" are to be found. In the field of health, consumers are not at all reliable allies in the struggle to contain costs. For they imagine themselves as potential patients or relatives of potential patients, and they are unwilling to restrain physicians or hospitals from purchasing expensive equipment. They also tend not to advocate closing down the unneeded hospital in their communities, for they wish to prevent the resultant loss of jobs and community status. Thus, goals that are widely deemed to be socially desirable (such as rational, cost-efficient health-delivery systems) will not necessarily be sought through consumer involvement.

In other words, those advocating participation as a goal in itself, as the essence and definition of democracy, and as an essential process in the fulfillment of the individual, need to realize that, like all important values, the values that

---

*These sentences are written in part with tongue in cheek, since there may not be an "objective measure" of what is the public welfare. But many of those who advocate citizens' participation are often also quite committed to the attainment of certain end-states which they believe to be "right": de-emphasizing high-cost, high-level technology in health care; establishing comprehensive secondary schools, etc.

motivate demands for participation may well collide with other
equally important, ultimate values. Some kind of balancing of
such values must be done. At times, central governments may
have to impose what is equitable, even if doing so limits the
sphere of self-determination.

Recent developments in the German health system are a
good example of the need for such balancing. The Cost
Containment Law (KVKG, 1977) certainly contains various
provisions which could be interpreted by the parties as
inimical to self-determination. For example, the remuneration
of doctors is to be determined through negotiations at the level
of the Land, not by the district. This provision prevents
physicians from playing off one district against another. But
it is a move toward greater centralization. Similarly, the
"point value" of services rendered by doctors will henceforth
be the same for all sickness funds, which means that the
Substitute Sickness Funds of white and blue collar employees
(Ersatzkassen) are no longer free to negotiate their own
schedules. This may well be excellent in terms of social
equity because it eliminates one way in which the majority of
blue collar workers are disadvantaged. But it restricts the
scope of what intermediate bodies can do independently. Also,
the new law prescribes new criteria which should guide
negotiations between Kassen and physicians in determining the
cost of physicians' services. The establishment of such
criteria can be viewed as a circumscription of the range of
participatory mechanisms. The criteria are designed to help
the consumer by linking growth of total health costs to the
growth of the total income of contributors. But however
desirable they may be, the criteria are nevertheless a
government prescription.

The new law also contains some innovations that increase
the scope of consumer participation. For example, the Kassen
will have somewhat more power in reviewing the cost
implications of how each physician conducts his or her
practice. They will also have more power to employ physicians
if the physicians' association fails to provide medical services
in a needy area. But it should be noted that these boosts to
the power of participatory mechanisms have been legislated
because they seem, on balance, the best way to achieve a
certain substantive goal. Participation is not being boosted
because it is in itself a long-term policy pursued for its own
sake.

It seems clear that participation as an end in itself will
usually be subordinated to an important substantive goal such
as the containment of health costs or the establishment of
comprehensive secondary schools. There is probably as much
willingness to sacrifice or to compromise participation for the
sake of other goals on the left as there is on the right. Although the left is ideologically more committed to participation

than the right, the left is also more committed than the right
to reaching certain substantive goals of equality.   Michels'
Iron Law of benevolent and enlightened oligarchy continues
to apply!

INCREASED CONTROL OF THE PROFESSIONS

The trend of slowing down, if not reversing, the increased
power of the professions may be as consistent a structural
political trend as the expansion of participation and the latter
may be viewed as a deliberately structured obverse and
corollary to the latter.   This assertion is deliberately couched
in relative terms because neither of these two trends is
dramatic.   Nor is either likely to become dramatic; certainly
the latter will not.
     The trend to check the power of the professions began in
the mid '70s.   Many of the laws and proposed laws in the area
of the social services in recent years have tended to constrain
in some way the economic and political powers of the
professions.   The entire problem of cost control in health
consists, essentially, of the question of whether physicians
and hospitals can be constrained.   Can they be prevented from
prescribing unnecessary diagnostic and therapeutic measures?
Can they be coordinated so that only one hospital in a certain
area will buy a certain piece of equipment or offer a certain
kind of specialized service?   Will it be possible to reduce the
number of beds and even the number of hospitals?   Will society
ultimately have to buy out physicians and hospitals to achieve
these ends, or can they be achieved through legislation and
regulation or through bargaining?   There are similar problems
in the area of education. The "tax revolt" that is attracting
such attention in western countries (although it, too, perhaps
is another exaggerated crisis) will have the effect of limiting
the freedom of the professionals and administrators in
education to design policy as they see fit.   The tax revolt is,
in part, a revolt against the immensity of expenditures.   But
if it is successful in reducing them, that will effectively
restrict the professions.   In education, it is a revolt against
professional educators who have introduced - according to the
public - too many "frills" and not enough "basics" in education.   In urban planning, it is the technical planners and the
politicians who are being constrained by new legislation.
     The professions are being attacked not only from outside,
but also from inside.   Their strength is being undermined
internally by oversupply.   Teachers are in oversupply in all
countries, largely because of sharply declining birth-rates.
Physicians are in oversupply in the United States and certainly
in Germany, where the annual supply will shortly exceed

demand by 60 percent. This oversupply will probably have a considerable impact on the incomes and the bargaining power of teachers and physicians.

As is usual in history, a variety of factors are acting together to produce the same result. It is therefore difficult to establish the exact significance of each. But the rapid rise in the economic and political status of the professions seems to have called forth several counterforces, all of which are working to restrict them. It has called forth an oversupply of professionals. It has called forth a consumer demand for participation in decision making in sectors in which the professions are active. It has called forth a reaction on the part of the state, from which the professions have asked too much. The state is helping to mobilize consumers to contain the professions.

18 The Agenda for Participation Research

Reinhard Oppermann

Demands for political participation in the form of direct citizen initiatives are increasing in all fields, but particularly in the areas of the environment, energy, health, education and local politics. In order for political scientists to analyze these new, powerful, and seemingly spontaneously engendered forces, some classification scheme and research agenda would be helpful.

Three types of participation starting from fundamentally different points can be distinguished. The first is the planning and decision-making participation which can be seen as input-oriented. It concentrates on the type and content of a decision. Most local and enviornmental participation initiatives fall into this category.

The second type of participation focuses on taking part in the realization of a decision itself, and can therefore be considered output-oriented. To this type belongs those kinds of participation which are always required in human services. This form of participation is most easily seen in the areas of health and education. The participation of the patient or student is taken for granted in these situations. Whether this can be considered in a politically participative framework depends on the amount of power in the hands of the subject - that is, whether it entails a responsible relationship or passive treatment.

The third type of participation is further from the classical concept of political participation: it no longer has to do with events or policies which were decided on by others (politicians) and administered by others (professionals). It is the takeover of the already realized programs of the professionals in the form of mutual self-help groups whose purpose is the revitalization of the social order. Examples of this type are new forms of communal living neighborhoods and women's groups. In economic terms, the concepts of "production" and "consumption" of services have no place in this form of participation. This is true of the second type to some extent also; however, in the third type it is broadened to include the rejection of the professionalized division of labor in favor of self-help.

While successes in the decision-making processes in the local, energy, and environmental areas can be seen and further pressures for more participation expected, participation in other areas has had only weak beginnings.

Demands for participation in some areas, particularly education, may be steered in a fixed and institutionalized framework and, in some countries, circumscribed by laws and mandatory regulations. Despite these and other constraints, there are no signs that demands for participation will diminish in the future.

Participation research at this time should focus on the following problems:

1. Which structural conditions produce barriers to participation? How can they be overcome and what chances do the various strategies and combinations of strategies have? Is there a danger that the "organized" participation will lead to a channeling of emancipated endeavors and how can this danger be countered? Is the combination of "organized" and "spontaneous" participation an unbearable contradiction or a condition for effectiveness in participation?

2. What socializing assumptions and consequences does participation have? Do groups with specific socioeconomic attitudes favor specific participation forms? Is there an explanation for successes in participation and their forms among certain classes?

3. What is the role of the scientist? Are they neutral researchers or engaged technical administrators? Wherein lie their possibilities as members of the technical-scientific intelligentsia and the middle class? What conflicts arise from belonging to this social position?

These three problem areas are not to be taken as complete or mutually exclusive. They simply illustrate the large group of problems still to explore. From the standpoint of knowledge we stand closer to the beginning than the end of participation research.

Index

Index

Foster/COMPARATIVE PUBLIC POLICY AND
    CITIZEN PARTICIPATION

Addendum to About the Contributors, p. 251

CHARLES R. FOSTER, a specialist in
bilingual education in the Department of
Education, serves concurrently as
Secretary-Treasurer of the Conference
on Atlantic Studies. He has taught at
Indiana University and the College of
William and Mary, and has published
extensively on German politics.

STEPHEN ARTNER, a 1978 graduate of the
 Johns Hopkins School of Advanced
 International Studies, is a visiting
 staff member of the Haus Rissen
International Institute for Politics
and Economics in Hamburg.

About the Contributors

DR. PRODOSH AICH teaches Sociology and Social Policy at the Carl-von-Ossietzky University in Oldenburg, West Germany.

DR. CHRISTA ALTENSTETTER is an Associate Professor in Political Science at the City University of New York and Research Fellow at the International Institute of Management in Berlin. She has taught at the University of Heidelberg, Syracuse University, American University, and the University of Kiel, Germany.

JOAN B. ARON was formerly an Associate Professor at the Graduate School of Public Administration, New York University. She came to Washington as a NASPAA fellow in 1976-77 and subsequently joined the staff of the Office of Policy Evaluation, U.S. Nuclear Regulatory Commission.

LAWRENCE D. BROWN, is currently Research Associate at the Brookings Institution in Washington, D. C.

WULF DREXLER, M.A., Dr. rer. soc., is a member of the planning staff of Oberstufen-Kolleg, where he has been since 1974 a teacher and curriculum researcher.

ADALBERT EVERS, Dr. rer. pol., born in 1948, is a scientific assistant at the Chair of Planning Theory, Department of Architecture of the Technical University of Aachen (FRG).

HEINO GALLAND is senior research associate for energy at the Battelle Institute in Frankfurt/M., West Germany.

MAURICE A. GARNIER is an associate professor of sociology at Indiana University.

RAIMUND KLAUSER, Diplom-Soziologe is involved in research in the fields of education and communication at the Institut fur Mediensoziologie/Medienpsychologie, Forschungs- und Entwicklungszentrum fur objektivierte Lehrund Lernverfahren (FEoLL) GmbH, Paderborn, West Germany.

HENRY A. LANDSBERGER is professor of sociology at the University of North Carolina in Chapel Hill, N.C. He lectures frequently in Europe on topics dealing with participation and the professions.

ROBERT A. LEVINE is currently Vice President of System Development Corporation; he is also the recipient of a German Marshall Fund grant for a pilot study of European program evaluation.

REINHARD OPPERMANN is currently the Director of the Task Force on Participation Research at the University of Bonn and Secretary of the Society for Participation Research.

VIRGINIA COHN PARKUM is Lecturer and Research Associate at the Yale University School of Organization and Management.

MICHAEL POLLAK is Research Associate at the Program on Science, Technology, and Society at Cornell University.

JUAN RODRIGUEZ-LORES, Dr. phil., is a scientific assistant at the Chair of Planning Theory, department for architecture of the Technical University of Aachen (FRG).

ROBERT H. SALISBURY is Professor of Political Science at Washington University.

UWE THAYSEN is professor of political science at the Luneburg Center of the University of Hamburg. He is also editor of the German Journal of Parliamentary Affairs and has written extensively on parliamentary reform as well as on current international affairs issues.

GORDON P. WHITAKER is Assistant Professor of Political Science at the University of North Carolina at Chapel Hill.

HORST ZILLESSEN is the director of the Social Science Research Institute of the Evangelical Churches of Germany, in Bochum.